Every Woman

Adapting to Mid-Life Change

H E L E N   D O A N Ph.D.

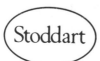

First published in 1987 by
Stoddart Publishing Co. Limited
34 Lesmill Road
Toronto, Canada
M3B 2T6

Canadian Cataloguing in Publication Data
Doan, Helen McKinnon, 1938-
    Every Woman: adapting to mid-life change

ISBN 0-7737-5079-7

1. Menopause.   2. Middle aged women — Health and hygiene.   I.
Title

RG186.D63 1987   612'.665   C87-093000-1

"Percentages of Women Reporting Symptoms by Age and Self Menopausal Status" reprinted by permission of Elsevier Science Publishing Co., Inc. from Frein Bernice Neugarten and Ruth Kraines, "Menopausal Symptoms in Women of Various Ages" in *Psychosomatic Medicine*, 1965 (2), 266-73. Copyright © 1965 by the American Psychosomatic Society, Inc.

"Hot Flash Diagram — Origin" and "Hot Flash Diagram —Spread" with accompanying text is reprinted *Menopause — Me and You* by permission of Dr. Ann Voda.

The "Hysterectomy Procedures" illustration and text is reprinted from *The New Our Bodies, Ourselves*, copyright © 1984 by The Boston Women's Health Book Collective. Reprinted by permission of Simon & Schuster, Inc.

Cover Design: Brant Cowie/Artplus
Cover Photograph: Mario Madau/Hot Shots

Printed in Canada

Contents

This book is dedicated to my parents, Helen and Harold Doan, for their many years of love and encouragement.

Preface

I have been interested in women's issues for many years, and started writing in this area a couple of years ago when Dr. Janice Morse and I wrote *Every Girl: Learning about Menstruation*. That book was written to provide a factual and sympathetic introduction to menstruation that would answer many of the questions girls had asked us, and hopefully meet their emotional needs.

As I began my reading to prepare for the first book, I became very interested in the topic of menopause and realized how little had been written about it. I started talking to a number of women, men and adolescents, and became aware of their ready acceptance of the many myths about menopause because they had few popular sources to turn to.

Both for personal reasons (I am a middle-aged perimenopausal woman), and to find out what actually had been written on the topic, I began an extensive search of the research literature and books that were available.

This book is a result of not only my literature search, but also I have included information collected from questionnaires and comments from interviews with women, men and adolescents.

My focus in this book is to stress that every woman is an individual and experiences life events, including menopause, in her own way. This message seems to me to be one that is not sufficiently stressed in many of the other materials I have read.

I would like to thank the many people who assisted me with their invaluable input, patience and time. Also, I very much appreciate the helpful comments from Lara, Bob and David.

Chapter One

Understanding Menopause

"Women were born to be in menopause! Menopause is as much a natural physiological characteristic of women as is menstruation, pregnancy,
and lactation."

Judith Golden, 1984

By the time she is middle-aged, every woman has gone through a
number of life stages. She has been an infant, preschooler, school-
aged child, adolescent, young adult and adult. Each of these stages
has its own set of life tasks, significant events, demands, and
challenges. Her ability to solve problems and her style of thinking
has changed. She has accumulated a number of life experiences
and memories. In spite of its importance as a distinct developmental stage, until relatively recently very little was written about
middle age. In fact, some writers describe middle age as having
been discovered only in the '70s and '80s, since so little research
was done on this topic until then.

For a woman, middle age brings with it many social and physical
changes. Her children may be leaving home, resulting in what has
been labeled the "empty nest syndrome." Her work and home
roles may be changing. Physically, not only may she start to notice
some differences in her appearance, but bodily changes are occurring that affect a woman's ability to bear children. *Menopause*, a
word derived from Greek, meaning monthly pause, is the term
used to describe this change in her reproductive capability. Just as
in every other stage of development, the major physical event, in
this case menopause, happens to every woman. However, each

woman's experiences, attitudes, knowledge, interpretation of and preparation for menopause varies. Each woman goes through the experience of menopause in her own way. Each has her own pattern of physical and emotional changes. Because menopause occurs in different ways for different women, understanding the range and type of variation can help each of us to put in better perspective our own experiences.

What is menopause?
There are many terms that are used to describe menopause. Also, to add to the confusion, different writers use the terms in slightly different ways. Accordingly, I thought it advisable to explain some of the main terms used in the literature on menopause.

While menopause is thought by many women as the whole time frame related to their changing reproductive capability, in scientific writing a woman is considered to be menopausal only when her menstrual periods have stopped completely for one to two years. The average age when menopause seems to occur is around 51 years. But the average range of age for menopause is between 45 and 55 years. The physical changes that are related to menopause are ongoing for about seven to ten years. Therefore, several terms are used to describe the different stages in the menopausal process:

- *Premenopausal* is a term that seems to be used in two ways. It is either used to refer to the time in a woman's life before any of the menopausal symptoms begin, or to describe the first three months when menstrual periods are starting to become irregular and some of the other early menopausal symptoms may be beginning.
- *Perimenopausal* is used by some to denote the period of time from when symptoms usually associated with menopause are starting to the time when menopause has occurred.
- *Postmenopausal* refers to the time after menopause has occurred, i.e., menstrual periods have ceased for one to two years.
- *Climacteric* is very often used synonymously with the term menopause. However, it has also been used broadly to reflect the entire series of changes that are taking place in middle age. More frequently, this term is used to describe the time when menopausal symptoms are occurring, which can also include the peri- and postmenopausal years.

In addition to the terms described above, there are many euphemisms for menopause, such as "change of life," "change of style," or "the change." These euphemisms are so general that they tend not to be very useful. However, an understanding of the other more specific terms can help women to clarify where they are in the menopausal process. Hopefully, this clarification can help middle-aged women understand themselves and the process of menopause better.

I asked a number of middle-aged women about symptoms that are typically related to menopause and where in the menopausal process they thought they were. Although the description of their symptoms indicated they were in the perimenopausal stage, several of these women felt they had not yet started the menopausal process. It is also interesting to note that the question I was most frequently asked by women was how they would know when they were starting menopause. Understanding that there are different stages in the menopausal process is a beginning of increasing self-awareness for the middle-aged woman.

Preparation for menopause

A few years ago Dr. Janice Morse and I collected information from a group of girls in grades seven and eight about their knowledge and feelings about menarche (or the beginning of menstruation). We were surprised by the finding that menarche and menstruation were, in many ways, still taboo topics, despite the many television advertisements which tended to suggest the opposite. We found attitudes towards menstruation of denial, embarrassment, and rejection when we tried to collect information that was intended to be helpful to young adolescents.

Although menstruation and menarche are still apparently taboo subjects, it is recognized that it is important to help young girls understand what they might expect with the changes in their bodies. As part of their school curriculum they see films and are given lectures on these topics. On the other hand, little information is generally available to women approaching menopause. Only recently have courses and support groups been available to help menopausal women, but they reach only a small percentage of women who could benefit from the information. When a group of women were asked *what they had heard and read about menopause*, the majority of them answered "not much." Other answers included:

- "I am not too interested."
- "Books are available on the subject in the doctor's office or hospital clinics."
- "*A Friend Indeed* publications are very informative and helpful."
- "My doctor answered my questions on menopause. I read about it in an encyclopedia."
- "Very little — not much empirical research has been done."
- "Some women are different from others."
- "A lot of jokes, mostly made by men."
- "A great deal of conflicting information and opinions."
- "I've heard people groan and say their mothers have gone crazy during menopause and are hard to live with."
- "I've got the impression that very little is known about menopause and that most women do not know what to expect."

As you can see, many women enter the menopausal years with little, no, or at best inadequate knowledge and accordingly with little, no, or at best inadequate preparation.

Why do so many women have so little information about menopause?

There seem to be many factors that account for this lack of information. For one thing, menopause and middle age are linked not only in a time frame, during the forties and fifties, but are viewed by many in potentially negative terms. "I'm not interested in the topic of menopause," was a frequent response from many women. Also, traditionally there have been many myths associated with menopause that have been accepted without question. In additon, knowledge about menopause may be affected by its newness as a concept. Until the last quarter of the nineteenth century, the word menopause did not exist in the English language. A century ago the average life expectancy was so low that the majority of European and American women did not live long enough to experience menopause.

Perhaps another factor that has determined the availability of information on menopause is that women have been too reticent and accepting of outside opinions and views on menopause.

Myths about menopause

Traditionally there has been a lack of information and little research about menopause and the topic has been considered taboo. As a result many myths about menopause have developed and persisted. Margaret Lock, a medical anthropologist, wrote in 1982 that "Menopause is a subject which has encouraged the development of mythologies since it is associated with much ambiguity and paradox."

Some of the myths are discussed by Janice Delaney, Mary Jane Lupton and Emily Toth. In their book, they give an example of a nineteenth-century physician who said that bad news could bring on an early menopause. Other causes of an early menopause were thought to be "irregular and unwomanly occupations, cooks from overeating, laundresses from being exposed to high temperatures." In addition, menopause was also attributed to alcohol, poverty, opium, typhoid and excessive sexual indulgence.

Not only were there myths about the cause of menopause but also about the effects of menopause on women. Again, Delaney, Lupton and Toth quote a Victorian gynecologist, Edward Tilt, who felt that with menopause there was a "gradual loss of feminine grace"; that women began to look masculine, thus "bones either stick out or are sunken in fat and their skin gets flabby and tweezers are sometimes required to remove stray hairs from the face." Tilt also reported that during menopause women were more susceptible to certain mental diseases, such as morbid irrationality, minor forms of hysteria, melancholia, impulses to drink spirits, steal, and murder.

You can see that these views of the menopausal woman are the basis of some of the contemporary myths surrounding menopause. Others you might hear today include:

• Menopausal women are all irritable and cranky.
• There is a decline in women's sexuality with menopause.
• Women who started menstruating early will experience menopause later in life.
• Women will go through menopause at the same time as their mothers did.
• All women going through menopause will experience debilitating symptoms.
• Women become much more masculine after menopause.
• Women who have a hysterectomy will go through menopause immediately after surgery.
• Some women become mentally ill due to menopause.
• Menopause makes women fat and causes graying and thinning hair, wrinkled skin, cracking fingernails, varicose veins, tooth decay, and more.

• After menopause women no longer produce any estrogen.

Unfortunately, these myths are the primary source of beliefs about menopause for some people. They can potentially affect the expectations, fears, and attitudes about menopause for the woman as well as members of her family and community. Thus, in some cases, a belief system is built up about menopause which does not recognize that each woman is an individual and is not based on scientific evidence.

Women's attitudes to menopause

Menopause is an event which all women will experience at some point and we all have our own feelings and attitudes about it. Sometimes, understanding other women's feelings can help us to put our own in perspective. Therefore, I asked a group of women a number of questions designed to ascertain their attitudes to different aspects of menopause.*

To get an overall view, the first question asked was *"What comes to mind when you hear the word menopause?"* In a group of women aged between 45 and 55, it did not seem to make much difference whether they were peri- or postmenopausal. However, their answers varied considerably.

• *To those relating to aging, menopause means:*
   – "Aging, death."
   – "The realization that I'm getting old."
   – "Being middle-aged."
   – "I'm getting older. No more menstruation."
• *To those stressing symptoms:*
   – "How will flushes affect my life?"
   – "Big change to your body."
   – "A time of adjustment."
   – "A terrible time of life in which one has to cope with hot flashes and depression."
• *To those focusing on changes in menstruation:*
   – "It's great not to have a period anymore."
   – "No more inconvenience of having periods."
   – "Freedom!"

---

* The answers of the women to the questions described through the book are from questionnaires administered to women who varied in age (fifty year olds; forty years olds; and twenty to thirty year olds) and economic class.

- *To those indicating limited change or lack of knowledge:*
  - "Another change in life like any other."
  - "Nothing much."
  - "Another stage in life."
  - "Nothing comes to mind."
  - "Nothing at all."
- *Positive and accepting answers:*
  - "Just another natural stage in life."
  - "An ending of one stage of life and the beginning of another stage."
- *Some were unsure:*
  - "Growth or curse?"
  - "I don't know if it's the beginning or end."

It is interesting that in this group of women where most were peri- or postmenopausal, there were several who had no opinion of menopause.

In the 40- to 45-year age group, these were some of the comments:

- "I'm a little nervous but it's not Panicville. It's just part of the aging process."
- "It's hot flashes, irregular menstruation, and sensitivity."
- "Aging, old."
- "Getting older Not having children."
- "Nothing at all."
- "No more periods."
- "Emotional problems."

Some examples of comments from the 20- to 39-year age group are:

- "Physical, hormonal body changes. Periods cease."
- "Not having to go through monthly periods."
- "Passing on to a new phase life."
- "A woman becomes moody because she can't accept the fact that she can no longer become pregnant."
- "An ending, loss of femininity, sadness."
- "Sexist men blame a woman's difficulties in middle age on menopause and don't try to understand her emotional/social problems."
- "Irritability and depression."

- "Personality changes."
- "Old age. Your body loses its ability to procreate. A certain part of you is taken away."

While the categories of responses in all groups were basically the same, and in fact very similar statements were made by women in each age group, the one noticeable difference was that women from the youngest group focused more on women's moods, irritability, and personality changes. That younger women tend to have more negative attitudes to menopause was also found by sociologist Dr. Bernice Neugarten and her colleagues.

Because it seems to be assumed by some that attitudes to menopause could be affected by *whether or not a woman wanted more children*, two groups of women were asked this question.

In the 40- to 55-year age group, only three women said yes, they would like more children if they could and were younger. The following comments are from the women who said no.

- "Even four is too much responsibility."
- "My children have been a great burden."
- "Past my prime. Other interests."
- "Always felt a person should only have the number they can cope with both financially and emotionally."
- "It is more worrisome today in everything in raising children."
- "We're satisfied with two and wouldn't want young children now."
- "I think we've done enough for the world population."
- "I want to develop my own interests now."
- "I enjoy my independence."
- "I now enjoy the freedom to come and go as I like. No more waking up at night and catering to small children."

It was interesting to me that many women in their twenties and thirties did not want to have any more children either:

- "Two is enough."
- "I don't care to go through the whole process of pregnancy, infancy, adolescence again. Three times is enough."
- "I want to provide my children with everything I can. I would have to compromise if I had more children. I also have other interests and enjoy being able to pursue them now."
- "Too organized, maybe too selfish with my time. Want to have the freedom. They might drive me up the wall."

- "Never. Children are a pain."

However, there were also many in this group who wanted to have or add to their family.

In interpreting these results, it is important to keep in mind that the groups who filled out these questionnaires were relatively small. However, if these results are representative, they do suggest that the older women were generally not concerned about having more children. While there may be a difference between not wanting children and not being able to have children, these results suggest that loss of fertility may not be a critical factor affecting women's attitude to menopause and for some, not being able to have more children could be seen as advantageous.

Women's attitudes to menopause were further examined by asking for opinions as to *whether or not menopause makes a difference in a woman's life.*

In the 40- to 55-year age range the women's comments suggested:

- *A positive change:*
  - "It's just for the better."
  - "Gives me more freedom."
- *A negative change:*
  - "I got hot flashes and was depressed for a time."
  - "Growing old, body sagging, more aches and pains."
- *No change or minor changes:*
  - "It's a minor moment on one's life — not a big deal."
  - "Not to my life."
  - "Aging makes the difference."
- *Temporary changes:*
  - "If anything, it makes everything more convenient. However, there may be some minor discomfort to deal with."
  - "At the transition period there are some difficulties. I hope these will disappear with time."
- *Individual reactions:*
  - "It all depends on the individual."
  - "Many women's sex lives get better because they don't have to fear pregnancy. But some women have trouble during coitus because the vagina is dryer. In general, one can stay as active after menopause as before."
- *No knowledge:*
  - "I don't know anything about it."
  - "I have no idea."

Of the women in the 20-30-year age group who felt that there would be changes with menopause, not one viewed the changes positively:

- *Negative changes:*
  - "Perhaps it changes the way she feels about herself during the time she is having menopause."
  - "Women have been socialized to believe that menopause is the beginning of the end."
  - "It signals the end of ability to create life. There must be a sense of loss."
  - "There are emotional and physical problems."
- *No change:*
  - "If she is supported through the experience, just like any other stressful time, there's no problem."
  - "Not unless she lets it."
- *Temporary changes:*
  - "Not after."
  - "Yes, at the time she is going through it, but later it all goes back to normal."

Since it is believed by some that menopause has an effect on a woman's appearance, I asked the women whether they associated menopause with changing physical appearance. In the women in the 40- and 55-year group, about half felt menopause had no effect on a woman's appearance. Those who felt there was a relationship, referred to:

- weight gain or loss
- the tension and stress that may change a woman's appearance
- waist thickening, hair graying and appearance of excess facial hair
- increased skin wrinkling.

One woman commented that "some women look and handle it much better than others." In the 20- and 30-year age group, the majority felt that menopause had little to do with physical appearance.

Since women may express a general view different from their impressions of how an event can affect their own lives, the women were asked *what they felt about their own change of life.* Again the older group, whether they were pre-, peri-, or post-menopausal, seemed to feel that menopause had little effect on their views. For example, some women who were in the peri-menopausal stage, and most of the women in their twenties and thirties, stated they felt nothing yet. However, some of the peri- and postmenopausal women's comments included:

- *Negative/ apprehensive*
  - "Life has been going downhill ever since I started the meno-pause. I'm depressed and the hot flashes bother me."
  - "I feel as though I am less healthy."
  - "I'm a little concerned about what kind of symptoms I will have."
  - "I'm a little bit apprehensive."
  - "I don't feel in control."
  - "I have some ambivalent feelings. I hope the symptoms are minimal and I'll be able to proceed with daily life in as normal a fashion as possible."
- *Positive*
  - "Just a part of the aging process but a very welcome change."
  - "I've accepted the fact that this is part of my life cycle."
  - "It seems to coincide with my most creative life period."
  - "I thought of it as a change of life, a new experience to deal with."
- *Neutral/acceptance*
  - "Not a big deal."
  - "It's just another stage in my life and I'll adjust to it."
  - "I'm accepting it. I don't think much of it."

While the group of women we questioned was relatively small, and it is difficult to know how representative they are and how honestly and thoroughly they answered the questions, it was clear that women's attitudes to menopause varied considerably.

- Some saw menopause as another developmental marker and for a few it was associated with growth.
- Others seemed to focus more on menopause as a medical condition.
- Some seemed more positive and others more negative.
- They differed in the degree to which they emphasized emotional problems.
- Some seemed aware of many issues relating to menopause; others demonstrated disinterest or lack of knowledge.
- More of the younger women seemed to be negative in their attitudes.

- They differed in the degree to which they associated physical changes of aging with menopause.
- Some seemed more concerned about the loss of femininity.

Thus, women not only experience menopause in their own individual way but their attitudes, expectations and concerns also varied. Understanding our own attitudes and expectations is important to us since it can affect:

- how we interpret symptoms (i.e., as a part of life or as debilitating);
- what we interpret as symptoms (i.e., if we believe all menopausal women are irritable, a perfectly normal reaction to an irritating situation could be misinterpreted as menopausal);
- what we expect in ourselves or other menopausal women. Psychologists point to what they call the self-fulfilling prophecy. Briefly, this means that our expectations (the prophecy) set in motion a behavioural sequence that ends up seeming to confirm (fulfill) our expectations. In other words, if you expect certain symptoms or reactions to occur at menopause, you may have them because of your expectations;
- how and what kind of treatment you may seek. For example, women who feel only "neurotic" women have symptoms may not seek medical help or psychological support at a time when it would be helpful for them.

In addition, there were many women who stated they were not aware of their feelings or had no opinions about menopause. Even if you separate out from this group those who did not feel like filling in the questionnaire, these findings indicate that there are a number of women with either limited information about menopause, or a lack of interest or who have not yet formed an opinion. What could be of more concern is that some of this group were describing symptoms that would suggest they were perimenopausal. If women actually feel that menopause is not a significant life event, you wonder how they would be prepared for changes if they occur, and whether these women might not be more open to myths or misinformation.

Negative attitudes about menopause could be based on a lack of information about what to expect, exposure to someone who had a particularly difficult time, myths about menopause, linking menopause with aging and becoming less attractive, or menopausal symptoms with which they are having difficulty dealing. Negative attitudes could also affect how symptoms, if they occur or are occurring, are interpreted.

Considering it might help to clarify women's attitudes to menopause, I asked a group of women about *their attitudes to menstruation.* The age of menarche in the group I questioned ranged from nine to 17 years. Interestingly, their comments on menstruation were very similar to those collected by Dr. Janice Morse and me from a group of grades seven and eight girls. Comments of the women, as expected, showed incredible variability. Some examples are:

- "Good."
- "I hate it. It is inconvenient, messy, debilitating and goes on forever."
- "I would like to be finished with it."
- "Nervous."
- "It's a bloody nuisance."
- "I felt comfortable. The only complication was the headache which sometimes lasted for the duration of the period."
- "Mostly I thought it was a nuisance but sometimes I related it to a feeling of femininity."
- "I have no feelings about it — perhaps a bit positive knowing that I am not pregnant."
- "I resent it. Why me? Why women? It's not fair. It's a pain."
- "I associate it with womanhood."

Despite the varied attitudes to menstruation, there seemed no simple relationship between attitudes to menstruation and attitudes to menopause. Some of the women who had positive views of menstruation also had positive attitudes to menopause. However, some did not. Also negative attitudes to menstruation were not necessarily associated with negative views of menopause.

It would seem reasonable that women's feelings of menopause would also be affected by the attitudes of their children, husbands, physicians and society in general.

Attitudes of husbands to their wives' menopause

> "For men, menopause is, of course, not an emo-
> tionally loaded issue: in many cases they consider the
> menopausal woman a rather comic figure. She is
> pictured with a red face, erratic moods and the
> ultimate parcel of female troubles. They may
> patronize her and pity her sad condition or
> wonder how they can aid the poor creature who
> is about to pass through a 'profound life crisis.' "
> *Dr. Weideger*

Very little research has been conducted to determine the attitude
of men to women in menopause. Kristi Dege and Jacqueline
Gretzinger examined the attitudes of family members to menopause in a small sample of families. With regard to husbands'
views of their wives' menopause they found:

• Some husbands were not willing to talk about "such things."
• Husbands generally held more negative views to menopause
  than their wives.
• Better-educated men were more positive in their attitudes.
• Husbands believed they could determine if a woman was
  menopausal by both physical and emotional symptoms. Mood
  changes and hot flashes were the most common symptoms,
  they felt.
• Most men said husbands give menopausal wives more understanding or stay out of their way and women give husbands a
  difficult time by being "ornery" and backing off.
• While women did not feel they treated their families differently
  during menopause, husbands felt that their wives did treat
  them differently.
• The husbands said they did not talk about menopause with
  their wives and learned about it from the media and family.

In spite of the men's confidence that they could identify menopausal symptoms, some researchers have found that husbands
have a general lack of knowledge about menopause and did not
know when changes occurred.

Using questionnaires, we asked a sample of *husbands about
their feelings about menopause*. The following are representative

of some of their views. Some were supportive and understanding, and others had difficulty dealing with their wives' menopause. For some men these problems may have been related to their associating their wives' menopause with their own aging. Others were bothered by the symptoms, i.e., if it affected their wife's sexuality or if they considered it made her irritable.

Most of the men associated menopause with more negative and medical terms such as:

• moodiness, increased sensitivity, irritability, crankiness
• a change of life with new moods and feelings
• a physiological and emotional experience
• aging and hot flashes.

Most of the men had very limited information about menopause, particularly in a more positive growth sense. Those who associated menopause with crankiness, moodiness or hot flashes usually had observed these symptoms in their wives or mothers. It could also be that men may become aware of menopause only when women inform them of their symptoms or when their symptoms become apparent, as with some hot flashes. Whatever the basis of their attitudes, if a husband's view of menopause is negative, it could affect his interpretation of his wife's behaviour as well as the way he treats her.

When we asked peri- and postmenopausal women *how their husbands perceive menopause* their answers included:

• "He's not thrilled."
• "He accepts it."
• "It's a natural process."
• "Nothing."
• "He feels concerned about growing old."
• "I don't know. We have never discussed it."
• "He seems to be fairly calm about it and deals with things as they happen."
• "He says there's nothing you can do about it. When it happens, it happens."
• "He associates it with growing old."

Some women felt that many husbands really don't know what their wives are going through with menopause. Others felt that husbands would be affected only if their wives are having serious health problems or feel an aversion to sex. There were others who felt a husband would be affected only if the wife "makes a big deal out of it". The husband's level of security and relationship with his wife were also suggested as important factors in determining his reactions. A more relaxed sex life was also a possible result of menopause, with both partners freed from the worry of pregnancy.

Children's attitudes to their mothers' menopause

A woman's adjustment to menopause could also be affected by her children's attitudes and reactions. Kristi Dege and Jacqueline Gretzinger also researched the attitudes of a group of children of menopausal women. They concluded:

- many of the adolescents had limited knowledge about menopause
- the children tended to have more negative attitudes to menopause than their mothers or fathers
- the children from better-educated families had more positive views
- the children from the lower educational background families associated menopause with a change in temperament; they felt their mothers became more irritable and grouchy
- the children from higher educational backgrounds focused more on the emotional and physical changes that were appropriate for a certain age
- children learned about menopause from their parents and peers.

In listening to adolescents talk about their mother's behaviour, it does not seem to be unusual for them to believe that if their mothers are "irritable," they are menopausal. One adolescent said, "All menopausal women are irritable and some became mentally disturbed. They get paranoid." It would appear that many adolescents pick up and accept society's myths about menopause. They seem to have a limited understanding of what menopause is or its effects. If the mother is negative about menopause, it could suggest that her children may not be supportive at a time when that support is needed.

We asked a group of peri- and postmenopausal women about their *perceptions of their children's attitudes to menopause*. Following are some of their answers.

- "They know nothing about it."
- "My children take it lightly. They accept it."
- "I've never discussed it with them."
- "It's a natural occurrence they have to learn to cope with."
- "They're sure that it will never happen to them."
- "They associate it with irritability, like 'being on the rag.' "

As can be seen, mothers and children do not tend to talk about menopause. Many children know very little about this important life event.

The fact that husbands and children know very little about menopause raises some concerns. Firstly, with whom do women share the menopausal experience? A group of women was asked about this. Some indicated that they felt it was a private matter and they spoke to no one about it; others shared their feelings with female friends; and a small proportion of the women sought advice from physicians. Secondly, what kind of support are women receiving from their families? Unless there is some understanding, it is unlikely that some women would be supported by their families while they are going through menopause. The third possible consequence of this lack of knowledge is that the attitudes of families can affect their interpretation of the woman's behaviour. As noted earlier, if the family assumes that menopause is accompanied by irritability, whenever a woman is irritable, whether it is an appropriate reaction or not, it could be interpreted as menopausal.

Drs. McKinlay and McKinlay wrote in 1973 that menopause is generally perceived in Western cultures as a "stigmatizing event in a woman's life marking the end of her social usefulness — procreation." It is interesting to note that based on some of the comments we received, this description is still appropriate today in some families.

Physicians' atttitudes to menopause

There have been two approaches used to examine physicians' attitudes to menopause: through the careful analysis of information presented in gynecology textbooks and by interviewing physicians. Margaret Lock helped to clarify some of the ambiguity women face when talking to physicians. Physicians, as Dr. Lock and several other researchers have reported, tend to focus on one of two different approaches to menopause. One of these approaches emphasizes a disease model, where menopause is related to a variety of physical and psychological complaints and where the primary treatment is drug oriented. The second approach stresses the relationship between menopausal symptoms and psychosocial factors that influence them, the "mind over matter" approach. Dr. Lock interviewed students, interns, and residents in obstetrics and gynecology at four teaching hospitals. From her interviews she set out several factors she felt influenced physicians' attitudes to menopause, such as the personality of her physician; the physician's attitude toward women; the age, sex and experience of the physician; and the physician's academic training.

It would seem to me that in addition to these points raised by Dr. Lock, other factors could influence the effectiveness of physicians in helping menopausal women.

• Some physicians by searching for a medical explanation to a menopausal woman's symptoms, may be missing other important causative factors. For example, a physician who sees depression in a patient as menopausal may be ignoring other, more important sources of the problem. It can be a real put-down for a woman who is experiencing a problem to be put off with "It's only menopausal."

• A physician who gives the impression that women should expect some problems associated with menopause may influence the number of symptoms a woman might report.

• The feeling of being confused yet rushed in an appointment with a physician can result in dissatisfaction for the woman.

We know that different physicians have different orientations to menopause which are translated into how they treat their menopausal patients and interpret their symptoms. Each of the approaches and models followed by different physicians is probably applicable and effective for some women and not to others. Every woman is an individual and menopause is an individual and complex experience. For some women it is probably more important to stress the medical or physical symptoms requiring predominantly medical treatment. For others, their ability to cope with what is happening in their lives is primary. Women may have similar symptoms springing from very different sources.

In 1983, Drs. Ann Voda and Mona Eliasson wrote,"The medical approach to explaining menopause appears to be inadequate for the majority of women, not only because in its present form it does not invite discussions, but because of the continuing emphasis by the medical establishment on menopause as a deficiency disease, one that needs to be treated."

Therefore, a physician's attitudes, manner, and knowledge can influence how effectively they can help an individual menopausal or perimenopausal woman. They could also have an influence on building expectations in premenopausal women and in encouraging or discouraging a discussion of the concerns of the pre-, peri- or postmenopausal woman. Some of the women with whom I spoke said that when they raised the topic of menopause with their physician, they were told they were not at that stage yet and the topic was quickly changed. These women expressed disappointment and felt their physicians would only talk about menopause seriously with them if their symptoms were of sufficient magnitude to require treatment.

Many statistics suggest that a number of women do not approach their physicians about the topic of menopause. For example, Dr. Patricia Kaufert, in 1980, reported the results of a Canadian study in which 44 percent of women between the ages of 40 and 60 had never raised the question of menopause with their physician. Eighty-three percent relied on books and magazines for information. Drs. Sonja McKinlay and Margot Jeffreys, in 1974, found that one in five women reporting hot flashes sought medical treatment. The group experiencing both acute physical discomfort and embarrassment were most likely to consult a physician. Drs. Rodney Meeks and G. William Bates stated that about 25 percent of women see a physician for menopausal symptoms. Dr. Johanna Perlmutter indicated similar findings, that is less than one third of women seek medical attention.

What these statistics suggest is that the medical profession may not be the most accessible and readily used source of information and support about menopause. One can only guess the many reasons why this is the case. These results, however, do suggest that it is important to be aware of your doctor's attitudes to menopause and to determine whether her or his approach is suitable for you.

Historical view of menopausal women

> "Woman is a pair of ovaries with a human being attached; whereon man is a human being furnished with a pair of testes."

The above quote was reported in Paula Weideger's 1977 book, *Menstruation and Menopause*. She used this as an example that our cultural heritage has dictated that woman is valued and valuable only as long as she can reproduce. This perception of women as primarily childbearers has historically been one of the factors that has affected how menopausal women are viewed as well as the quantity and type of research and writing about menopause over the years. Menopause has also been, as menstruation has, a taboo topic that has been of relatively little interest.

Historically, the primary themes of those writing about menopause have related to:

- whether menopause is seen as a deficiency disease or is more a psychological phenomenon;
- whether the focus should be on medical care (the medicalization of menopause) or on supporting and encouraging developmental growth;
- whether menopause is seen as a time of loss or growth;
- the importance of maintaining youthful qualities;
- whether the postmenopausal years are a time of waiting to die or developing new skills and enjoying new freedom.

Involved in discussions of these issues have been physicians, nurses, anthropologists, psychologists, sociologists, psychoanalysts, feminists, and writers. Reading through the material that describes the historical views of menopause, it is easy to see the origin of myths surrounding the subject.

Drs. Haspels and van Keep refer to a book by Gardanne, written in 1816, as the first book devoted entirely to the female climacteric. In this book, Gardanne described the cessation of menstruation and named the syndrome *la Menespausie*. Drs. Haspels and van Keep also noted that until the French Revolution there was almost complete disinterest of the medical profession in climacteric-related problems. Part of this lack of interest is explained by the low age-expectancy for women and the use by women of midwives rather than doctors.

The lack of knowledge about menopause, and thus the type of treatment given, is reflected in the description in Delaney, Lupton, and Toth's book about menopause treatment by Victorian gynecologist Edward Tilt. Dr. Tilt's treatment to London women for menopause was mineral water, morphine, syrup of iron and potassium, exercises, travelling, bandaging of limbs, sedatives, and abdominal belts. But the preferred treatment at the time was bleeding effected by placing leeches behind the ears. The surgical removal of the uterus and the ovaries was invented by Robert Battey in 1872. The early surgery was carried out without any anaesthetic.

Not all Victorians perceived menopause as negative. Suffragist Eliza Fornham in the 1860s saw menopause as a time of "secret joy," of "spiritual growth of super-exaltation."

Psychoanalysts contributed to the portrayal of menopause as a negative time, a time of loss. They formed their opinions primarily through observation of "neurotic" clinical patients. However, they generalized their theories to all women. Delaney, Lupton, and Toth described the view of menopause by the founder of psychoanalysis, Sigmund Freud. They noted that Freud felt that menopause was a time when previously undisturbed women could become "quarrelsome, obstinate, petty and stingy, show typical sadistic and anal-erotic features they did not show before."

Helene Deutsch, in *The Psychology of Women, vol. II*, published in 1944, followed the views of Freud and said "At the moment when expulsion of ova from the ovary ceases all organic processes devoted to the service of the species stop. Woman has ended her existence as a bearer of new future, and has reached her natural end — her partial death as a servant of the species. She is now engaged in an active struggle against her decline."

One feels in reading some of these writings that women at menopause, like salmon having struggled to lay their eggs, have reached the end of their life cycle. What writers like Helene Deutsch did was to turn the information collected from a small number of non-representative women into a theory of female adjustment that encouraged negative views of menopause. Some of these views remain today.

Barbara Ehrenreich and Deidre English, in *For Her Own Good*, described that at the turn of the century, women could only look forward to menopause portrayed in the medical literature as a terminal illness, the death of the woman in a woman.

This loss of femininity has been a theme of many books describing menopausal women. For example, David Reuben, in his popular book, *Everything You Always Wanted to Know About Sex*, stated: "As the estrogen is shut off, a woman comes as close as she can to being a man. Increased facial hair, deepened voice, obesity, and the decline of breasts and female genitalia all contribute to a masculine appearance. Coarsened features, enlargement of the clitoris, and gradual baldness complete the picture. Not really a man but no longer a functional woman, these individuals live in a world of intersex."

My reaction in reading David Reuben's book was that I really did not want to know his conception of everything, primarily because his representation of the menopausal woman was so inaccurate and endorsed many misconceptions. Concepts such as "no longer a woman" and "living decay" have been used by writers to describe the menopausal woman. It is easy to see the basis of the caricature of the menopausal woman, with her irritability, red face, and perception of being of limited value to society.

Dr. Robert Wilson, in 1966, wrote a book titled *Feminine Forever*, which had an incredible effect on the treatment of menopausal women. Dr. Wilson accepted the misconceptions of the time and suggested estrogen replacement therapy as necessary treatment.

- "Instead of being condemned to witness the death of their own womanhood during what should be their best years, they will remain fully feminine — physically and emotionally — for as long as they live."
- "Menopause must at last be recognized as a major medical problem in modern society. Women, after all, have the right to remain women. They should not have to live as sexual neuters for half their lives."
- ". . . the traditional attitude of many physicians, who simply refuse to recognize menopause for what it is — a serious, painful, and often crippling disease."
- "Enlightened physicians who see menopause for what it is — a preventable and curable deficiency disease — are still in the minority."
- "Her husband, her family, and her entire relationship to the outside world are affected almost as strongly as her own body."

Dr. Wilson's view of menopausal woman was probably based on his observations of clinical patients who came to him with their problems. Unfortunately, he generalized his findings to all menopausal women and reinforced previous misconceptions. Not only did he describe menopausal women in derogatory terms but he told women and other physicians that in order to remain feminine forever women should take estrogen replacement therapy. He felt that menopause was unnecessary and could be prevented entirely. "Younger women need never experience it. And older woman can in most cases be assured almost complete recovery from their symptoms." Estrogen therapy was, therefore, recommended for women prior to the development of any symptoms and for those who already were experiencing problems associated with menopause. He even felt that "youthful appearance and vigorous energy can be retained through estrogen therapy for decades beyond the customary age of menopausal decline."

As a result of the popularity of Dr. Wilson's book, estrogen became a standard treatment for many menopausal women. In the 1970s medical researchers began to find a relationship between uterine cancer and estrogen therapy. As this finding gained credence, some women and physicians began to question whether estrogen was a necessary treatment for all women. Gena Corea, however, in the 1977 book *The Hidden Malpractice: How American medicine treats women as patients and professionals*, referred to a report of Jane Brody of the *New York Times*, who made spot checks around the United States and found that each of the 12 physicians she called said reports did not prove that estrogen directly caused cancer and, in the absence of proof, no drastic changes were warranted. In spite of Jane Brody's results, it seems that more women began to be more directly involved in their treatment and the widespread use of estrogen therapy lessened. Drs. Haspels and van Keep commented that 15 to 20 years after Wilson's book "some 10 percent of all American women in the postmenopausal take estrogens with the purpose to prevent a number of the phenomenon of aging because they want to achieve the American dream of eternal youth."

The feminist movement that gained strength in the '60s and '70s played a major and active role in advancing women's awareness of issues. Particularly, it influenced the attitudes and treatment of menopause in the following ways:

• Feminist writers, for example Rosetta Reitz, author of *Menopause: A Positive Approach*, gave women an alternative to the interpretation of menopause as a deficiency disease and stressed instead the positive, growth-oriented aspects.
• Feminist researchers have encouraged, developed, and carried out research which has helped to clarify some of the factors that affect a woman's menopausal experience.
• Information has been provided for women about their bodies generally. For example, a book written by the Boston Women's

Health Book Collective, *Our Bodies, Ourselves*, was published in 1973. A revised version, *The New Our Bodies, Ourselves*, came out in 1984. It covers topics ranging from "Taking Care of Ourselves" (food, body image, alcohol, etc.) to "Relationships and Sexuality", "Controlling Our Fertility", and "Childbearing". The increasing awareness and importance of menopause to women is evident in the expanded treatment in the revised edition.

- Health centers, journals, and support groups have been developed to inform and assist women with issues related to their bodies.
- Feminist writers and groups have encouraged women to take an active role in decisions affecting them.

In the '80s there is more research being conducted into the topics relating to menopause. Anthropologists are studying cross-cultural comparisons of the menopausal experience to help us to understand women's reactions to menopause in different parts of the world. Psychologists and sociologists are conducting research to determine some of the factors that may influence an individual woman's menopausal experience. Physicians and nurses are researching menopausal symptoms and treatment. It is interesting to note that some of the physicians still describe menopause as a deficiency disease, while others focus more on developmental and psychological factors. Many of the issues that were important historically are still being discussed. Now, however, a much wider perspective is being taken.

Where are we now? Those interested in the topic of menopause have considerably more information and support available to them than did earlier generations. However, there is still much to learn. In addition, there are different approaches to meet the varied needs of women. For example, the writings of some of the feminists would be encouraging and helpful to many women. On the other hand, for many women the emphasis on a medical interpretation is more appropriate. Each woman approaches and experiences menopause in her own way.

Chapter Two

Middle Age

"Age cannot wither her, nor custom stale
her infinite variety."
Antony and Cleopatra (2.2.238.239)

In the play, Enobarbus is describing the young Cleopatra in a way
that implies a strength of appearance and personality that is
timeless. This quotation raises some of the myths of aging yet at
the same time denies that they need exist. But I like the notion
that changes associated with aging can be viewed in a positive
way, recognizing that physical changes may occur but that there
can also be growth, increasing relaxation, and developing of inner
strength and relationships.

Many years ago I was visiting with a woman in her fifties. Her
20-year-old nephew, whom she had not seen for a few years, was
also there. On the first night of his visit, as we sat down to dinner,
the young man looked at his aunt and, no doubt trying to impress
her, said, "You're looking very young." "Why would I want to be
young? I'm happy where I am," she replied rather quickly. The
young man had not impressed his aunt but I was certainly
impressed with her. My friend was truly enjoying her status as a
middle-aged woman who was settled in her career and lifestyle.

Unfortunately, there are many women who do not have as
positive a view of aging as this friend of mine. Some are apprehensive about their changing physical appearance. "Why can't my
mother see herself as a beautiful woman for her age instead of
focusing on her wrinkles and thinking they are ugly?" some children say. Some approach aging with concern about their job prospects, thinking "How can I compare myself with young people

who are aggressive and have knowledge of so much more than I?" And others focus on their possible problems with finding a mate/ friend: "Why would anyone be interested in me when there are so many beautiful young women around?"

In trying to understand a woman's attitudes to menopause, it is necessary to separate her attitudes and concerns to being middle-aged. As mentioned earlier, menopause usually occurs between the ages of 45 and 55 years. Middle age is usually defined as the age between 40 and 60 or 65 years (unless you use the definition, once stated vehemently by my daughter when she was about eight years old, that middle age starts at 60):

> "Until recently, midlife seemed little more than a way sta-tion between youth and old age, not worthy of much thought or discussion. Then, suddenly, it became a crisis — a moment of high drama when we supposedly struggle with the recognition of our own impending mortality, when life's unfinished tasks loom large and painfully in our consciousness. In fact, it's neither way station nor crisis, but a stage in the life cycle like any other — a time of life with its own dilemmas, its own tasks, its own pleasures, its own pains."

It would be nice to be able to be as philosophical about middle age as Lillian Rubin has been in this quotation from her book *Women Of a Certain Age*. It is clear, however that there is a wide range of opinions about middle age among women:

- "I'm going to be 40 in two weeks. I've told everyone not to remember my birthday."
- "I'm already in middle age and I haven't accomplished what I planned by now."
- "Forty was like any other birthday. I kind of expected to feel terrible. So many of my friends had but I know I haven't accomplished everything I want but I am more comfortable with myself."
- "Why is it that when men turn 50 we celebrate their accomp-lishments? When women turn 50 they hide."

When some women were asked *what they felt were the major changes that occurred during middle age*, many expressed positive attitudes towards the changes:

- "Middle age means maturity, security, finding a place to spend the rest of my life, and realizing I'm responsible for my own fate."
- "It's having more time to pursue the things I enjoy and less responsibility at home. More social life."
- "I've got more active children, they're growing up. Therefore there's more time to be spent *with* them, not like before, just cleaning up, but dealing with their emotional needs."
- "No periods. No premenstrual tension. Less stress."
- "I want to discover myself, who I am, what I want to do with *my* life and how I want to relate to my fellow humans. It's a search for meaning and self-actualization."

On the other hand, some felt there would be no changes:

- "I don't forsee any major changes. What is middle age anyway — 35, 45, 55 or 65?"
- "Nothing other than normal physical changes."
- "I don't feel there will be any major changes. I will always try to be the way I am now — young."

There was a small number of women who focussed more on their concerns about middle age.

- "I'm concerned about adapting from working full-time to not working at all."
- "I worry about my parents."
- "Less energy. Restricted activities."
- "I think more about death."
- "It brings loss of hair, a pot belly, and worries about maintaining one's health."

There are many factors that help to determine how women will feel about middle age. Some of these relate to societal views of aging women and others to our personal experiences. Perhaps a discussion of some of these issues will assist in clarifying your own position.

The middle-aged woman of today will have to deal with some of the same situations as her predecesors.

Changing physical appearance
Susan Sontag, in her 1972 article, "The Double Standard of Aging," wrote:

- "Getting older is less profoundly wounding for a man, for in addition to the propaganda for youth that puts both men and women on the defensive as they age, there is a double standard about aging that denounces women with special severity."
- "For most women, aging means a humiliating process of gradual sexual disqualification."
- "Women are at a disadvantage because their sexual candidacy depends on meeting certain much stricter 'conditions' related to looks and age."
- "Men are 'allowed' to look older without sexual penalty. . . .The single standard of beauty for women dictates that they must go on having clear skin. Every wrinkle, every line, every gray hair is a defeat."

While we may or may not agree with Susan Sontag's view, it is clear that the middle-aged woman is constantly being bombarded with products that promise her renewed youth. Walking through any department store, one is struck by the number of products to colour graying hair, smooth out facial and neck wrinkles, keep aging hands looking young.

Sociologist Dr. Judith Posner, in an article published in 1984 on aging and advertising, commented, "Popular advertising does much to reflect and aggravate the particular stigma of aging for women in our society. In fact, a majority of aging-related products are specifically directed at the female vis-a-vis the male."

These advertisements tell us among other things, that their products can

- through an age-smoothing skincare, achieve "the complexion to shoot for — firm, fresh and crystalline-pure"
- give us a "radiant and youthful look"
- get rid of "impaired beauty" caused by wrinkles
- get rid of "unsightly" gray hair.

Life events and middle age

Children with different scholastic or vocational goals
Mothers and their children can differ in their academic and vocational goals and these differences seem most apparent at the time the mother is middle-aged. For example:

- the mother valuing homework and good grades; the adolescent valuing friends and long telephone conversations that interfere with homework.

- the mother encouraging her daughter or son to attend university; the adolescent or young adult not wanting to attend university or dropping out prior to graduation.
- the mother wanting her child to have a professional position; the young person being disillusioned with school and not interested in a profession.

The degree of stress these differences can create for a middle-aged woman may be related to the degree to which she identifies with the "success" of her children.

Children leaving home
What some call the "empty nest syndrome," or children leaving home, has been suggested by some to be a major factor affecting middle-aged women. However, it is clear that women deal with their children leaving in very different ways:

- Some have a problem with their children leaving home and feel "lonely and worried if they are alright"; "left out"; "very upset"; "a little empty"; "disappointed" or "very sad."
- Others are pleased, "happy for them"; "relieved when the first two left and will be ecstatic when the last one leaves"; "very happy"; "glad they are growing up and feel able to cope"; "proud of her accomplishments"; "happy to be free of so many day-to-day responsibilities, more money for self and spouse."
- "It's all in the process of life. They have to leave some day. We will visit each other and create a more loving relationship."
- Still others have mixed feelings and are "sorry to see her leave but looking forward to more freedom"; "in some respects good and others sad"; "glad they are growing up and lonely they are gone."

Their reactions may be related to their relationship with their children ("Relieved. There is so much conflict at home."); husband ("I am looking forward to having more time alone with my husband" and "My husband and I have grown apart over the last few years. I'll feel very sad when my daughter leaves."); and whether or not they have other interests ("I am planning to find outside interests to fill any void that might occur."):

If a woman has perceived herself as primarily a mother, having her children leave may precipitate a severe reaction. On the other hand, if a woman has viewed herself as both a wife and mother, she can often enjoy the time she has with her husband alone, knowing her children are growing and developing and she is still an important person to them, even though her contact and influence may be less direct. Some researchers have suggested that parents who have the least satisfaction with each other are more affected by the departure of their children.

Divorce

For some middle-aged women, divorce is a serious problem because they do not feel they are likely to have other close relationships. Other women are pleased to end an unsuccessful marriage and to develop and pursue their own interests.

Widowhood

Widowhood brings an incredible sense of loneliness to some women. They discuss losing friends who were close to them when they were part of a couple or there being many times when singles are not welcome at social gatherings. Also, some find it difficult to find new companions.

Other potential areas of difficulty for a middle-aged woman include:

- concern about her own or her husband's health
- financial responsibility and caring for aging parents
- her husband's feelings about being middle-aged and how he handles it
- retirement
- changing patterns and expectations of sexuality
- the relationship with her husband (e.g., her husband may be working long hours to reach the pinnacle of his career and therefore be more distant and preoccupied)
- her success in meeting, or being able to meet, her expectations in her career plans.

In addition to the factors just described, the middle-aged mother of today faces some potential issues that were not as important for her mother.

- Adolescence is a time for dealing with identity, sexuality, boy/ girlfriend relationships, and vocational plans. Teenagers have been well-known for handling these tasks by becoming more irritable or difficult. However, the world of the teenager today is, generally speaking, very different from that of a generation ago. Young adolescents are forced to deal with questions about sexuality, drugs, and alcohol that use very different from those which their parents faced.

• Sexuality and contraception are issues few parents can avoid.

• Many teenagers have selected a style of music with which they identify. Each style of music has associated with it a style of dress and behavior. For example, many parents find it extremely difficult to deal with their children wearing second-hand black clothes, with old-fashioned jewellery, dark make-up, black-dyed hair, and haircuts that seem extreme. I was told the story of one mother who, when her daughter appeared with her hair not only standing upright in a "punk" hairstyle but also with streaks of pink, green and blue, went to her own hairdresser and, after checking that the dye would wash out, had her own hair dyed green, pink and blue and put into a "punk" style. When she went home, her daughter, seeing her mother's hairstyle, immediately changed her own back to her usual style. While not all of us are as brave or as much of a risk taker as that mother, many are faced with similar problems.

• Another problem I hear of frequently is from middle-aged parents who are having difficulty with their teenagers about their curfew. "Juice bars" or discotheques operate late into the night, which may place considerable pressure on the young person to stay out late.

• There are other, more serious problems which parents may have to face. For example, the number of teenager pregnancies has increased, as have teenage suicide rates.

• In terms of having a feeling of parental competence and respect from their children, many parents now feel they have very little "power" in their relationships with their teenagers, who will walk out on them and go and live with a friend if they do not like their parents' decisions.

Thus, middle age is potentially a time of many role changes and decisions. For some, it is a time of stock taking. Some feel effective and competent and at the peak of their power and for others just coping is a difficult process.

Tasks of middle age

Psychologists have discussed the tasks that middle-aged people must accomplish to feel satisfied with their lives. Dr. Robert Havighurst describes some of these:

- achieving adult civic and social responsiblity
- establishing and maintaining an economic standard of living
- developing adult leisure-time activities
- assisting teenage children to become responsible and happy adults
- relating oneself to one's spouse as a person
- accepting and adjusting to the physiological changes of middle age
- adjusting to aging parents.

Erik Erikson, a psychoanalyst, saw middle age as a time when the issues were between what he called "generativity" and "self absorption." By generativity, Erikson was referring to taking as active a role in giving and responding to the needs of the next generation, integrating work with family life and increasing one's cultural potential on a greater scale. Some writers question whether Erikson's stages apply to women. Women, they feel, have been nurturing long enough and now need to become more aggressive and focus more attention on their own goals.

Gail Sheehy, in her book *Passages*, also described the goals of midlife. She stated that the midlife period is a time of a full-out authenticity crisis, when each individual has to come to terms with her ideal self and actual self. But the crisis makes sweeping changes in personality possible. There is a need at this time to re-examine the self, to forge an identity that is authentically ours. From childhood identification with our parents we carry along the most primitive layer of imaginary protection which shields us from facing our own absolute separateness. She sees midlife as a time of re-evaluation of our life and a period of restabilization.

Menopause, then, occurs at a time when women's roles are changing. Each woman experiences not only physical changes in her own way but she will also have different experiences with which to cope.

Chapter Three

Your Body and You

What's happening to my body during menopause?
In order to help you understand what is happening to your body
during menopause, it seems advisable to review the process of
menstruating. Menstrual periods occur because of a complicated
interplay between our brains and our ovaries. Menstruation is the
result of a complex feedback system between the hypothalamus
and pituitary glands in our brains and our ovaries.

The hypothamalus is the region in the lower, frontal area of the
brain that, according to the *Bantam Medical Dictionary*, "contains
several important centers controlling body temperature, thirst,
hunger and eating, water balance and sexual function. It is also
closely connected with emotional activity for sleep and functions
as a center for the integration of hormonal and autonomic nervous activity." The pituitary gland is a pea-sized organ located
slightly below the hypothalamus. It is also called the master endo-
crine gland. It secretes several hormones that affect many parts of
our body. The secretion of these different hormones is regulated
by specific hormone-releasing factors which are produced in the
hypothalamus. Finally, the ovary, also according to the *Bantam's
Medical Dictionary*, is "the main female reproductive organ,
which produces ova (egg cells) and steroid hormones in a regular
cycle in response to hormones from the pituitary gland. There are
two ovaries, situated in the lower abdomen, one on each side of
the womb. Each ovary contains numerous follicles, within which
the ova develop but only a small proportion of them reach maturity."* During menstruation, blood and fragments of the uterine

---

*According to Drs. Michael Soules and William Bremner, the following
represent the number of egg cells present at each stage of development: the fetus
has 2,000,000; at birth 1,000,000; 6-15 years 440,000; 16-25 years 160,000; 26-35
years 60,000 and 36-45 30,000. While the absolute number of egg cells is slightly
different from study to study, it is clear that with age the number decreases.

lining are discharged from the vagina at intervals of approximately 28 days. Dr. Lucienne Lanson, in a book titled *From Woman to Woman*, indicated menstruation "implies the occurrence of two elaborate and precisely timed events prior to actual bleeding: (a) ovulation (release of an egg by the ovary), and (b) specific changes in the tissue lining of the uterine cavity as a result of that ovulation." However, not all menstrual periods involve ovulation. Some are "anovular," which means that menstruation has occurred without the previous release of an egg cell from the ovary.

There is, then, a delicate balance between the functioning of the hypothalamus, pituitary gland, and ovaries, in which there is a complex interplay between these different glands during the menstrual cycle. Some researchers believe that the hypothalamus responds to lower levels of estrogen. The hypothalamus releases a hormone, the gonadotrophin releasing hormone, that acts on the pituitary gland causing it to secrete two other hormones, the follicle stimulating hormone (FSH) and the lutenizing hormone (LH). These hormones affect the ovary differently and the timing of their release is carefully integrated. When released, the follicle stimulating hormone stimulates certain follicles (which are sacs or glands in the ovary which contain the egg cells or ova) in the ovary. The stimulated follicles become enlarged and produce estrogen.

It might be helpful here to digress briefly to tell you a little about estrogen. Estrogen is the hormone that promotes the functioning of the female sex organs. According to Drs. Soules and Bremner, there are three naturally occuring estrogens: estrone, estradiol, and estriol. Estradiol is the principal estrogen in the reproductive years both in quantity and potency. Estrone is a quantitatively important estrogen but less potent than estradiol. Estriol is a weak estrogen which is primarily produced as a metabolic product of the other two estrogens.

To return to the follicle stimulating hormone: it affects the immature follicles in such a way that some of them develop into dominant ones and migrate to the surface of the ovary (it could be one or more than one that change this way). As this occurs, estrogen is produced which stimulates the lining of the uterus, called the endometrium. The uterus begins to thicken as new cells grow. As the estrogen level starts to increase, the level of follicle stimulating hormone starts to decline. At this time the pituitary gland secretes lutenizing hormone, which ruptures the follicle and releases the egg. This is called ovulation. After ovulation, the ruptured follicle continues to produce not only estrogen but also progesterone. Progesterone, therefore, is present at ovulation and prepares the tissue of the uterus lining to receive a fertilized egg. The ruptured follicle becomes the *corpus luteum*, or yellow body. If there is no fertilization, the *corpus luteum* starts to shrink and levels of estrogen and progesterone gradually decline. The endometrium starts to disintegrate and menstruation occurs. With menstruation there is a drop in the levels of estrogen and progesterone, which signals the pituitary gland, which in turn starts the cycle again by producing the follicle stimulating hormone.

The egg travels from the ovary to the fallopian tubes and then to the uterus. If it is fertilized, there is feedback to the *corpus luteum*, which during the first two or three months of pregnancy continues to produce estrogen and progesterone, which are vital for the growth of the fertilized egg. After this the *corpus luteum* ceases to function and there is no further activity within the ovaries. According to Dr. Lanson, they "are literally in a state of suspended animation — no stimulation of follicles, no ovulation and no hormone production. Estrogen and progesterone, as well as other hormones associated with pregnancy are derived exclusively from fetal and placental sources."

With menopause there is a change in the functioning of the hypothalamic/pituitary/ovarian balance. For some women this process takes a period of years, for others, their menstrual periods will stop suddenly. Rosetta Reitz, in her book, *Menopause: A Positive Approach*, summarized the literature indicating that cessation of menses can occur in one of three ways: abruptly, gradually, and irregularly.

"Abruptly, means the period stops and there are no more menstrual periods. . . . Gradually means the period changes by slowly diminishing in amount and length of flow. This is the result of the gradual shift in hormonal balance. . . . A woman may hardly notice the gradual change, for it may occur over a period of time lasting anywhere from six months to three years. . . . The periods may become scant and she may skip a period; or the periods may gradually become irregular but with cyclic regularity. That is, one, two, three, four or more periods may be skipped, but when the flow appears again, it is in the structure of the cycle. . . . Irregularity is by far the most common way for menstruation to cease. The menstrual pattern becomes increasingly irregular. The flow may vary from heavy to scant without any apparent pattern. The number of days of flow may also become irregular. The length of time between periods may become irregular too. A single month or many months may be skipped or periods can occur within a shorter range of time than the usual cycle. It is not unusual to go for a whole year without any periods and then get one or more."

It is not clear what starts the process of menopause. Some of the researchers believe that it starts with a decreased sensitivity of the hypothalamus gland to estrogen levels; others assume that the ovaries decline first. Whatever the cause, there are several gradual changes that occur:

- *In the ovaries*
  - The number of ovarian follicles declines, therefore the main source of ovarian estrogen is lessened.
  - The ovaries become less responsive to pituitary hormone stimulation.
  - The type of tissue within the ovary changes, with less space devoted to functional follicles and more to supportive tissue.
  - The ovary tends to lose weight as structural changes within it occur.
  - As the main source of ovarian estrogen declines, there is eventually no ovulation, no formation of a *corpus luteum*, no production of progesterone, and no cyclic ovarian function.
  - Some of the follicles that mature become atrophic, which means they cannot be fertilized and do not produce as much estrogen.
  - There is a decrease in the viability of the *corpus luteum*, again with its implications for hormone production and ability to release an egg to become fertilized.
  - With aging there is an increase in the number of anovular cycles. However, some women continue to ovulate over a longer period than others.

- *In the hypothalamus and pituitary glands*
  - Some researchers believe the hypothalamus becomes decreasingly responsive to the feedback from the levels of estrogen.
  - As the level of estrogen declines, higher levels of follicle stimulating hormone and lutenizing hormone are required in an attempt to compensate for this change.

– Dr. Lanson described the changing balance between the hypothalamus/pituitary/ovarian functioning in this way:

"Try imagining for a moment a giant seesaw. On one side are the pituitary hormones (FSH and LH); and on the other are the ovarian hormones (estrogen and progesterone). For thirty-five years or so, regular menstrual cycles have depended upon the pituitary and ovarian hormones seesaw-ing back and forth in perfect harmony. Thus, each time the ovaries produced more estrogen, down went the level of pituitary hormones; when the ovaries put out less estrogen, up went the level of pituitary hormones.

"But now as the ovaries begin slowing down during the menopausal years, this beautifully balanced seesaw is thrown off kilter. With less and less estrogen being produced by the ovaries, the pituitary responds by pouring out five, ten or even a hundred times more FSH than ever before in a des-perate attempt to stir up the sluggish ovaries. In short order the hypothalamus also becomes affected."

As you can see, the hormones involved in menstruation differ in the amount produced and their origin. There is another way in which the hormones are controlled. Through what is called the metabolic clearance rate, the hormones are processed at different rates. Drs. Winnifred Cutler and Celso-Ramón Garcia indicated that while there is still some disagreement about this, there may be a decline in the metabolic clearance rate of the hormones such as estrogen.

Although with menopause there is a decrease in the production of estrogen, it does not mean that your body no longer produces any estrogen. Dr. Lanson noted that for some women a few follicles can continue to produce some estrogen for five to ten years. Each woman has her own pattern of change. Drs. Soules and Bremner commented that as menopause occurs the estradiol levels drop to less than 10 percent of the premenopausal level, while estrone becomes the quantitatively dominant estrogen, around 33 percent of that during the reproductive period.

In postmenopausal women, the primary source of estrogen comes from the conversion of an androgen into estrogen. The androgen (called androstenedione) is produced both by the ovar-ies and adrenal glands and then released into the bloodstream. Some of the hormone is then picked up and converted into estro-gen in the fat deposits of the body. The amount of estrogen produced by this conversion varies from woman to woman. The heavier woman would by this process tend to produce more estrogen. However, the level of estrogen produced will always be lower than it was prior to menopause.

However can I know if I'm starting menopause?

It is very difficult to identify exactly when menopause is beginning. It is most likely that the first sign you will notice is a change in your menstrual flow. As explained earlier, the change can be either abrupt, gradual, or irregular. Some women start having hot flashes before they notice their periods becoming irregular.

Because the change in menstrual flow will probably be the first indicator, it is wise to keep a regular chart of your monthly periods as you approach the usual age of menopause. This chart will help you better understand your own body and perhaps be more comfortable with changes as they occur. It will also provide your physician with more exact information.

There are several ways in which you can keep track of your menstrual cycles. The information that would be most helpful for you would be the frequency of your periods, their duration, and the intensity of the flow. You can keep track of this material either by recording the information on a calendar or in a small notebook. If you use a calendar, just mark the first day of your period with a number 1, and each day of flow with a consecutive number; e.g., if you flowed for five days, you would mark a 1 on the first day, a 2 on the second, up to a 5 on the fifth day. Then you would continue numbering the days until you start to menstruate again. In addition, you could record if the flow was heavy (H), medium (M), or light (L). While these evaluations will be very subjective, they will provide you with information about changes in your cycles. Remember that the most important part of keeping track of your periods in this way is that it helps you become more aware of your own body and any changes that are occurring.

Is there a way my doctor could know if I'm menopausal?

There are several ways in which your physician could get an estimate of your menopausal status:

- The most common method used is through the menstrual history. Keep in mind, however, that there are several factors that can affect your menstrual flow, such as stress, extreme dieting, etc.

- You can measure estrogen levels through blood tests. Again, in interpreting this information you should know that estrogen levels normally change over a period of time and that to be accurate you should have several readings.
- Blood tests can also be used to record the levels of follicle stimulating hormone, lutenizing hormone and progesterone.
- You can measure the levels of pregnanediol, which is formed during the metabolism of progesterone, from urine tests.
- If a smear is taken from the upper vagina during a Pap test, it can be examined microscopically to determine the type of cells present. In the vagina there are three types of cells superficial, intermediate, and parabasal. These cell types differ in their degree of maturity and differentiation. The superficial cells are the most mature, the parabasal the least. At different stages in a woman's development the ratio of the different types of cells changes. With menopause, the number of superficial cells declines.

To understand any of the results from these medical tests, keep in mind that the interpretation of these tests is not always easy, as hormones can fluctuate over time.

Chapter Four

Menopausal Symptoms

"I feel that my friends and I view the menopause
as another of life's cycles. We do not dread it or
anticipate it. However, we hear stories of physical
annoyances! Overall, I believe that well-adjusted,
confident women will continue to be so, and that
women who are depressed and self-conscious will
be that way during and after menopause as well."

"There seems to be some women who do suffer
real discomfort during this period due to physically caused factors. How large is this group?
There are also a good number of women who
seem to suffer from vague symptoms (hysteri-
cal?). Are they the ones who do not really suffer
from menopause, but rather who have not come
to terms with aging? Maybe there is an overlap
and a need to sort out which variables belong to
the one or the other category."

These two quotations are typical responses to questions about
menopausal symptoms. They are representative of the questions,
knowledge, and concerns of women in their mid- to late forties
who are approaching menopause. There were many other questions and symptoms described by women ranging in age from 19
to 55. The following are summaries of their comments:

- There was a belief by some that women have control over how they react to their menopausal symptoms. "Some don't seem to give in to menopause." "Some can take it in their stride, others are ill a great deal or depressed or feel very sorry for themselves."
- Women of all ages described patterns of symptoms associated with menopause, such as hot flashes, irritability, forgetfulness, skin crawling, dizzy spells. Perhaps in trying to evaluate if one is menopausal, it would be important to take into consideration one's history of symptoms.
- Some of the patterns of symptoms described seemed to be related to stressful events in the woman's life, financial problems, for example. However, some women who noted minimal stress had the same symptoms as those who noted high stress.
- The women were generally not aware of when they were in the perimenopausal stage. Many would describe themselves as premenopausal when they were in the appropriate age group for menopause, had irregular periods over the past few months, and other symptoms characteristic of menopause.
- Some were aware that not all women have symptoms during menopause. "Some women have no problems or discomfort and handle the situation quite well. Others are uncomfortable and confused and don't do well."
- The women felt very differently about the onset of menopausal symptoms. For example, some talked about the end of fertility, being less of a woman, the end of health, physical discomfort, and nervous upset. Others were positive and talked about symptoms being a minor incident to be dealt with, knowing they would end soon.
- Some women who had had hysterectomies without both ovaries being removed had faulty assumptions about menopause. They assumed that they would not experience any menopausal symptoms because they had gone through menopause as a result of the operation.
- Some women stated that symptoms were most difficult when they became obvious. "The visible symptoms worried me, like sweating in public."
- Some of the women in their forties commented they felt embarrassed that they were so uninformed. Younger women generally noted a lack of interest in the topic. In fact, the women most apparently interested in menopausal symptoms

were those who were presently symptomatic. If this group is representative, their comments would suggest that many women become menopausal with limited information about what to expect.

• Many of the women were still confused about the myths and realities of menopause. Many were unsure of what to expect or what their symptoms meant. For example,

– A twenty-five year old woman wrote "Having suffered with premenstrual syndrome, menopause is scary. I wish people were more educated on the topic so the stigma could be erased."

– A 39-year-old woman who while still having regular periods had several menopausal symptoms, (hot flashes), did not realize there was a possibility she was perimenopausal and noted, "I will deal with the symptoms when they happen and get medical help if necessary."

– A 44-year-old perimenopausal woman stated that, "It is a bit frightening sometimes. You feel like life has passed you by and you are not 20 anymore."

– A 46-year-old perimenopausal woman stated that, "Women had to survive the stereotypes."

The women raised some excellent questions about menopausal symptoms, which follow.

Why do some women sail through menopause and others suffer debilitating symptoms ?
Every woman enters and experiences menopause in her own unique way. This uniqueness is expressed in the number, pattern duration, intensity, and frequency of symptoms she has.

Several researchers have statistically evaluated how many women experience symptoms and of these which are mild, moderate, or severe. The statistics vary slightly from study to study but they give us a general idea of what can be expected. It would appear that somewhere between 10 and 20 percent of women tend to experience a symptom-free menopause, at least in terms of the symptoms they reported. Around 75 to 85 percent have mild or moderate problems. Another 10 to 15 percent seem to have severe symptoms. Thus only a relatively small percentage of women have what would be considered debilitating symptoms. While trying to understand when symptoms become debilitating it is necessary to look at their duration and frequency. For example, more severe symptoms may be less overwhelming if they only last for a short period of time. For some women, menopausal symptoms last for a relatively short period of time while for others the symptoms may last over a period of years. Although our knowledge of menopause is constantly increasing, we still do not know exactly what causes the symptoms, to what extent they are due to changes in estrogen levels, brain chemistry or interactions of these.

The degree to which symptoms may be debilitating to a woman could be affected also by the woman's attitudes, expectations, and preparation for menopause. Role models such as mothers, sisters or aunts who have experienced menopause, her own menstrual history, support within the home or community, and ability to cope with unpredictability could also affect how a woman reacts to symptoms.

Women's attitudes to menopausal symptoms
On the basis of discussions with many women, it becomes clear that some do have debilitating symptoms. However, there are other women who describe very similar symptoms but who do not feel that they are debilitating. While it is very difficult to compare symptoms, it is possible that part of the effect of a symptom might relate to how women perceive it. We do know from a great deal of psychological research that while the stimulus presented to a group of people may be the same, their interpretation of the effect of the stimulus may differ. With regards to menopausal symptoms, women may interpret them differently because:

- different women may have different thresholds for tolerating symptoms and discomfort;
- the same symptoms, e.g., irritability or depression, could have different causes, which could affect how the woman deals with the symptom. (For example, if a menopausal woman is depressed because she is having marital problems with her husband and her children are leaving home, she would probably be affected differently than a woman whose depression seems more directly a result of menopause and who has a good relationship at home.);
- some women may be generally more vulnerable to stress and, therefore, menopause, perhaps in combination with other factors in the environment, may cause more problems;
- women differ in how significant they feel any physical or emotional symptom is;

- women's general attitude to menopause and aging may differ and may make it more or less acceptable to have any symptoms;
- some women are better at coping with their symptoms than others, thus, affecting their interpretation of the symptom.(For example, some women stated that during menopause they felt irritable but that they were very busy and just did not let it bother them.);
- some women have better support systems which may help them to perceive symptoms as less debilitating;
- some women found the symptoms very debilitating because they were not sure how long they would last. Some even said that if they knew the symptoms would be over in a certain period of time they would feel better.

Preparation for menopause

Very few women seem to be prepared for menopause. And, in some ways, it is a difficult event for which to be prepared because of the individual nature of women's experiences. Most women report that they discuss menopause with their physician only after the symptoms occur. Of the women who completed question-naires, none of the 20- and 30- year olds, five of the 40-year olds and two of the 50-year olds felt they were prepared for meno-pause. It seems reasonable that the more prepared a woman is for menopause, the easier it would be to cope, even with menopausal symptoms.

Role models

There is a great deal of psychological research that shows we learn by observing others. For many women the only preparation they have for menopause is observation of the reactions of other older women, their mothers, sisters, or aunts. Expectations, fears and coping strategies can be transferred from one woman to another. Just imagine how differently you would feel if an important woman in your life had any of the following experiences with menopause:

- "My mother was very sick and lost weight."
- "My mother's, sister's and aunt's experiences with menopause were all bad. They all had hysterectomies early."
- "My sister-in-law is having very uncomfortable hot flashes."
- "My mother was extremely depressed and demanding while menopausal. It was a very difficult time in her life."

Compare these comments to the following.

- "Nothing at all."
- "All the women I know seemed to handle menopause very well with no major problems."
- "My mother's experience with menopause was easy."
- "My mother had no problems whatsoever."
- "My mother had hot flashes and we would all laugh sometimes when her face became rather red but she did not seem to be bothered by it. There were really no differences in how she was before, during or after menopause."
- "My mother had some physical symptoms but she was very accepting of them."
- "Menopause was very uneventful."

You can see that a woman's expectations for menopause could be very different depending on, for example, her mother's attitudes and ability to cope with menopause. She could also interpret her symptoms differently.

Ability to cope with unpredictability
There are many aspects of the menopausal process that can be unpredictable; the way menstruation ends, the type of symptoms the woman has or the duration of the symptoms. As stated earlier, Rosetta Reitz noted there were three ways that menstruation could stop: abruptly, gradually or irregularly. Of these, irregularly is by far the most common way. Irregularity is experienced in the menstrual pattern, the amount of flow, and the number of days of flow. Therefore, there are many ways in which menstruation can become unpredictable. This means that women sometimes have to be prepared for a menstrual period at any time and when it does not occur, some may be concerned about pregnancy or problems with their health.

Women who are more comfortable with structure and timetables may find it difficult to cope with the unpredictability of menopause. Women also vary in their coping strategies for dealing with unpredictability. For example, some may be concerned and upset if something unpredictable happens, while others may not be so concerned but may see a doctor to check out the changes.

Women may differ both in their knowledge about menstrual changes during menopause and in their ability to cope with the unpredictability. It may also be that for some women who are already stressed for other reasons, this irregularity may interact with any menopausal symptom to make this period seem debilitating.

Research findings

There is also a body of research that may help us to understand why symptoms associated with menopause may be more or less debilitating.

- Some researchers suggest that women who undergo artificial menopause (with the surgical removal of the uterus, fallopian tubes, cervix and ovaries) are more likely to experience more menopausal symptoms. Dr. Lauitzen, in 1975, noted that women who have their ovaries removed often experience hot flashes and sweats about four to six days after surgery.
- Findings are inconsistent with regard to the connection between dysmenorrhea (or painful menstrual periods), pre-menstrual syndrome, premenstrual tension, and menopausal symptoms.
- There seems to be no relationship between the age of meno-pause and menarche (the beginning of the menstrual periods), although Drs. Cutler and Garcia reported that women who entered menarche later reported fewer menopausal complaints than those who entered earlier.
- Women who smoke are more likely to experience menopause earlier.
- There is no clear relationship between the use of the birth control pill and menopause, although a study by Dr. Treloar, in 1981, demonstrated that women who used estrogen in the five years prior to menopause were more likely to experience menopause one to two years later.
- There is no clear connection between the number of pregnan-cies and early or late menopause.
- Bernice Neugarten and Gunhild Hagestad, in an article pub-lished in 1976, argued that life course transitions were not ordinarily traumatic if they occurred on time because they were rehearsed and anticipated. Mary Clare Lennon found that menopause was a less distressing event when it occurred in midlife (45-54 years of age). She argued that it may be that when menopause occurs within the appropriate time more social support, advice, and information may be available.
- Drs. Greene and Cooke found that life stress was the more powerful influence on the elevation of menopausal symptoms.

They suggested that the reason for this finding may be that women who are experiencing a high degree of stress may be predisposed to act adversely to a high degree of life stress.

• Nancy Fugate Woods argued for a multicausative, multiple effect of factors on menopausal symptoms. She listed a number of variables which have been related to biological distress. These factors included rapidity of hormonal fluctuations, menopausal status, estrogen production in the ovaries, and the history of dysmenorrhea. She stated there was a positive association between the number of symptoms anticipated and life satisfaction for white but not black women. Attitude to femininity (i.e., the more "feminine", the more problems), to childbearing, and fertility (women who did not want to have more children had a more positive experience) were also related to distress. Other factors like marital status, social class, and income were inconsistently related. She reported that women with social support seemed to respond more positively.

• Drs. Cutler and Garcia suggested that nulliparity (having no pregnancies) and unmarried status were associated with fewer complaints. A last pregnancy after 40 years of age gave women more protection. It should be noted, however, that not all studies have found these results.

Thus, the research literature suggests a number of factors that may be related to menopausal distress. However, there is no easy answer. The menopausal process is very complex and is affected by physiological, psychological, cultural, and environmental variables.

What is a menopausal syndrome ?
Some researchers believe that there are a variety of physical and psychological symptoms that are found sufficiently often to form a menopausal syndrome. According to Nancy Fugate Woods, a menopausal syndrome assumes a deficiency model; that is, that a pattern of symptoms is related to estrogen deficiency.

Another approach to menopausal symptomatology simply considers combinations of symptoms as a symptom complex. This indicates that there are a variety of symptoms, such as hot flashes, night sweats, insomnia, and headaches, that seem to be frequently present in women at menopause. However, this analysis assumes that there could be multiple causes for these symptoms.

What symptoms might I have when I'm menopausal?
There has been a tremendous amount written about the symptoms that are commonly associated with menopause. From this material, several conclusions can be drawn.

• There is great variation in the type, frequency, duration, and pattern of symptoms among women. For some, symptoms related to menopause are apparent before the cessation of menstrual periods. For others, the symptoms coincide with menopause. There are other symptoms that do not appear until several years later. There is also a group of women who remain symptom-free.

• Symptoms have been related to every body system: vasomotor (pertaining to the muscular walls of the blood vessels), cardiovascular, metabolic, sensory, digestive, skeletal, muscular, glandular, and central nervous system.

• Several investigators have organized the symptoms into three main types: somatic (e.g., hot flashes), psychomotor (e.g., tiredness), and psychological (e.g., depression). Dr. Greene pointed out that these three categories of symptoms are independent and, therefore, the occurrence of one does not mean the natural occurrence of others.

• There is an incredible variety of symptoms that have been associated with menopause. As you can see as you read the list, it is very difficult to separate out the symptoms that are related to age and those that are exclusively associated with menopause. For example, Hilary Maddox summarized the symptoms as follows: hot flashes, sweating, chills, loss of sleep, headaches, disruptions of bladder causing more frequent urination, dizziness, vertigo (sometimes accompanied by nausea or loss of appetite), diarrhea and/or constipation, muscle aches and pains, increase in blood pressure, increased vaginal discharge and/or infection, irregular periods with varying amounts of flow, bloating, and flooding. In addition, others have described changes in libido, palpitations, psychological symptoms with anxiety, depression, mood swings, emotionality and irritability, increased risk of coronary artery disease, atherosclerosis, and hypertension. While still other writers focus on changes in the skin and subcutaneous tissue (loss of elasticity in the tissues and skin), and mucosal linings of the body (the linings in the eyes, nose, mouth, and vagina undergo atrophy or become drier). Stress incontinence and osteoporosis have also been associated with menopause, as has, what is called, formication or a feeling of insects crawling over the skin.

- In a 1965 study by Bernic Neugarten and Ruth Kraines, it is clear that many of the symptoms do not relate solely to menopause.

TABLE I
Percentages of Women Reporting Symptoms by Age and Self Menopausal Status

Symptoms	13—18	20—29	30—44	Pre-or post-meno-pausal	45—54 Meno-pausal
Somatic					
Hot flushes†	29°	6°	24°	28°	68
Cold flushes†	19	6°	13°	16°	32
Weight gain	47	30°	40°	41°	61
Flooding	23°	22°	40	24°	51
Rheumatic pains†	7°	6°	33	46	49
Aches in back of neck and skull	27°	26°	36	34	46
Cold hands and feet	53	40	36	31	42
Numbness and tingling†	18°	14°	27	37	37
Breast pains	20°	28	31	10°	37
Constipation	28	50	36	24	37
Diarrhea	29	46	25	20	24
Skin crawls†	11	6°	5°	3°	15
Psychosomatic					
Tired feelings†	82	96	84	71	88
Headaches†	77	80	76	47°	71
Pounding of the heart†	29°	22°	31	36	44
Dizzy spells†	39	30	36	36	40
Blind spots before the eyes	12	2°	9	14	22
Psychologic					
Irritable and nervous†	76°	90	82	71°	92
Feel blue and depressed†	79	88	62°	56°	78
Forgetfulness	49	52	51	60	64
Excitable	68	64	51	47	59
Trouble sleeping	49	44	45	40	51
Can't concentrate	65	52	56	46	49
Crying spells	57	50	36	38	42
Feeling of suffocation	9°	0°	13°	2°	29
Worry about body	35	20	19	24	24
Feeling of fright or panic	35	20	18	22	22
Worry about nervous breakdown	10	6	11	7	5

Figures in *italics* indicate the group reporting highest incidence of the symptoms.
° Significantly lower than menopausal mean (p < .05)
† Symptoms comprising the BMI.

As can be seen in this table, the greatest number of psychological symptoms are reported by adolescents. Neugarten and Kraines note the somatic and psychosomatic symptoms are reported most often by the menopausal women. As mentioned earlier, our results were similar to those of Dr. Llewellyn-Jones; there is a similarity of symptoms at all ages.

- Dr. Janet McArthur, in a 1981 article, described the early, intermediate and late menopausal symptoms as follows:

Early symptoms
- menstrual disorders
- hot flashes with sweating, especially at night
- minor nervous symptoms, such as difficulty with decisions and concentration, anxiety, loss of confidence, feelings of unworthiness and forgetfulness. (Although, she commented that these problems appeared to be more related to age than to menopausal status, as I am sure many of us will quickly agree.)

Intermediate symptoms
- atrophy of the estrogen-dependent tissues in the vagina which can be related to vaginitis (inflammation of the vagina which can be associated with irritation, discharge and pain in passing urine) which can cause painful sexual intercourse (dyspareunia)
- stress incontinence (involuntary loss of urine that occurs when laughing, coughing, or sneezing)
- dryness in the other areas susceptible to estrogen withdrawal such as the skin, gums, nose and mouth
- inelasticity of the urethra
- the connective tissue and muscular supports of the vagina, urethra and rectum undergo atrophy
- later on in the menopausal process, the vulva (or the external part of the female genitals), uterus, and ovaries shrink in size.

Late Symptoms
- osteoporosis (loss of bone mass)
- perhaps coronary arteriosclerotic heart disease.

Reading a list of symptoms like this one can be rather frightening. Other comments about menopause can help put these into perspective.

- Reading a list of the potential symptoms associated with menopause was described by many of the women as discouraging: "When I read about the symptoms of menopause, it made me feel frightened, old, and discouraged." For these women, it is important to emphasize that the symptoms are merely a list of what has been associated with menopause. Not all women will have all these symptoms. For the ones who do, most will find them minimal in nature. There are also possible treatments that can help women if they have problems.

- It is very difficult to separate some of the symptoms of menopause from reactions to other physical or life events. There can be other physical causes related to changes in the ovaries, or depression could be the result of many different stressful conditions.

- While hot flashes, vaginal changes, and changes in menstrual patterns have been linked directly to the lowering levels of estrogen, other symptoms can not be so easily explained.

- Many women are rather surprised and concerned when they exhibit symptoms which they previously thought of as "neurotic" and that they would never experience such as depression. "I have always been a happy, and what I considered to be a stable, normal person and all of a sudden I found myself quite depressed."

- In listening to discussions of postmenopausal women, one of the things they found comforting was to know that many of the symptoms were transitory. Also the symptoms such as hot flashes decrease over time in intensity and associated discomfort.

- For some women, menopause may cause minimal physical changes but it may trigger a reaction to other problems. If a woman is having problems with her marriage and has lost interest in sex, signs of the menopause may be exaggerated in order to remove her from sexual contact with her husband. Or if a woman has, for other reasons, a poor concept of self, any menopausal symptom will reinforce her feelings of being old and unattractive. For these women it is necessary to separate these reactions and deal with the real source of the problems.

- It is important to keep in mind that there are multiple causes for any symptom. The use of menopause as a simple explanation can potentially interfere with exploring the actual cause of the problem. "Since I'm in the right age range for menopause I assumed my fatigue, irritability, and depression were simply a result of this condition. However, my husband encouraged me to go to my doctor and I found out I had a thyroid problem. Since my thyroid problem has been treated most of my problems have disappeared."

- For some women, their family and friends are more encouraging and sympathetic to them when they are not well. Menopause could, therefore, be a time when having symptoms is positively reinforced. Psychologists call this "secondary gain" of symptoms.

- The relationship between stress and menopausal symptoms was examined by Dr. Susan Ballinger in 1975. She found that patients who had significantly higher scores on stress showed no difference in the percentage of women who had hot flashes or vaginal atrophy (dryness). The high-stressed women did, however, have higher clinician-rated depression and perceived similar symptoms as causing more distress.

- One woman commented that she felt that it was almost better to not read about menopause because it may make women look for symptoms that are not there and if a woman is suggestive, it may create symptoms. There are studies that show that some people handle medical problems better, the better informed they are. For others, they feel better not knowing.

While this section has been on symptoms, I am in no way trying to place the primary emphasis in this area. The emphasis when thinking about menopause should be not on the symptoms, but on the fact that it is a natural part of women's maturing. The menopausal years can lead to a new and exciting phase in a woman's life.

Information on symptoms in this book is to provide women with sufficient knowledge to help their understanding of their own symptoms. It would be helpful, therefore, to describe in detail some of the more frequently encountered symptoms.

Depression

According to many researchers, there is no evidence to suggest that menopause precipitates a depressive illness. However, some women do experience feelings of depression during the menopausal years.

There is some very interesting research investigating the interpretation of depression at menopause. At the moment the cause of depression is still controversial. Some authors suggest that the altering estrogen levels are related. Others focus more on a psychological intepretation or relate the depression to the lack of sleep associated with night sweats. Still others, for example Dr. McArthur, feel that "depressive symptoms in the 40- to 50-year decade are sometimes wrongly attributed to the menopause when, in fact, they are indicative of the syndrome of premenstrual tension." Drs. Meeks and Bates postulated a very interesting theory of depression: they feel that the menopausal depression may be related to the effects of estrogen concentration on the chemistry of the brain.

It is most likely that there are many reasons for depression in menopausal women. What we do know is that women who have never experienced depression prior to menopause may have some problems at this time. We also know that previously "normal," "stable" women can be depressed during menopause and that the depression usually does not last for a long period of time.

Stress and urge urinary incontinence

Stress urinary incontinence refers to the leaking of urine or the inability to retain urine during a sneeze, cough, jog, or laugh. Urge incontinence is the leaking of small quantities of urine prior to the act of urinating. Dr. Perlmutter commented that the amount involved could be from a few drops to "copious fluid at one's feet".

According to Drs. Meeks and Bates, stress urinary incontinence occurs in about 15 percent of both pre- and postmenopausal women. On the other hand, Dr. Ann Voda, in her research on hot flashes, found that about 75 percent of the women studied experienced the leaking of urine.

Stress and urge incontinence are thought to be due to the relaxation of the tissues and muscles in the bladder and there are exercises that can be used to strengthen this area. Also according to Dr. Voda, in her book *Menopause: Me and You*, "If you are obese, loss of weight will help. If you have a chronic cough due to smoking, stop smoking. Getting rid of the cough will help. Use of vaginal creams containing estrogen may reduce both stress and urge incontinence, but such creams should be used with caution and discrimination."

The exercise that is used to improve stress and urge incontinence is called the Kegal exercise. This exercise can be used either when you are urinating or when you are just sitting and have some time to practice. If you are sitting on the toilet, after starting to urinate you stop and hold your urine for about five seconds. Keep repeating this until your bladder is empty. Ann Voda stressed that it is important not to do this exercise the first time you urinate in the morning. She also noted that there should be about five to ten contractions per session, with relaxation for about three to five seconds in between. If you are not on the toilet you can sit anywhere and gradually tighten the muscles in the vaginal area, hold them for the few seconds and then slowly release them.

Vaginal atrophy

"I went to the doctor and he told me I had vaginal atrophy. I thought it was going to fall off."

This woman's comments reflect clearly two things: one is that one of the common menopausal symptoms is not understood by many women, and the words can produce fear and concern; secondly, it reflects a poor communication between a woman and her physician.

Vaginal atrophy is the term used to describe the changes in the vagina that can occur due to menopause. The vaginal walls may become thinner and the vaginal lubrication is lessened. Estelle Fuchs reported that vaginal atrophy is severe in 20 to 25 percent of women within a ten-year period after menopause and in about 37 percent after menopause. On the other hand, Judith Golden felt that approximately 50 percent of women have some vaginal changes.

The reason for the changes is that the vagina is highly sensitive to the levels of estrogen. Some women report that changes in vaginal lubriation produce painful intercourse and burning and painful urination. It seems that women who continue to have a regular sex life, either through sexual activity with a partner or through masturbation, reduce the likelihood of vaginal atrophy. Estrogen creams applied locally in the vagina are the usual treatment. Estrogen applied in the vaginal area will be absorbed into the general circulation, therefore great care should be taken if this treatment is used. If you are at high risk regarding the use of estrogens generally, you must not use this type of therapy at all.

Lubrication problems during sexual intercourse may be solved by more foreplay or the use of oil or jelly, such as baby oil, Vaseline or KY jelly.

Migraine headaches

Dr. Robert Greenblatt and his colleagues defined migraine headaches as being of slow onset, lasting four to 24 hours, precipitated by tension, alcohol or smoking, with symptoms such as an aura, nausea, and vomiting. For some women the onset of migraines coincides with the year of menarche. Also, some have migraines that are menstrually-related attacks. The other types are vascular or tension related. Since there is some evidence that some women experience a remission during pregnancy, and for some the head-aches are menstrually related, it seems that there is a relationship between migraines and sex steroids. It is not surprising, therefore, that some women have problems with migraines during menopause.

Hot flashes
One of the most frequently reported symptoms associated with menopause is the hot flash. Hot flashes have been described both as a physical and subjective event. Subjectively women experience a feeling of heat within or on the body, especially in the face and neck areas. This feeling of warmth has a point of origin and spreads over the body. It is often followed by a chill and perspiration.

There are characteristic physical symptoms associated with the hot flash. During a hot flash the internal temperature of the body decreases, the external temperature increases on the fingers, toes and cheeks, and the heart rate, at the onset of the flash, increases. Research has revealed the following:

- The time of onset is variable; that is, it may occur months or years before the final menstrual period.
- It may or may not be visible to others. If it is visible it will be seen as splotchy, red coloration of the face and neck.
- Not all women experience hot flashes. The percentage of women reported to have hot flashes differs from study to study. However, the data suggest that somewhere around 75 percent of menopausal women have hot flashes, although the range is from 10 to 89 percent. It is interesting that some researchers report a cultural difference in the frequency of hot flashes. For example, Dr. Margaret Lock did not find the women in her study in Japan reporting any hot flashes.
- Some women feel embarrassed, others do not.
- Some women experience acute discomfort. In a 1974 study, Drs. McKinley and Jefferys found that about 49 percent of those with hot flashes said they felt acute physical discomfort, with or without embarrassment, although 20 percent felt embarrassment but not acute discomfort.
- The number of hot flashes women experience varies through the day from infrequently (four or five times) to frequently (every half hour) throughout the day and night.
- Each woman has her own individual pattern of a hot flash with

a point of origin, and pattern of spread throughout areas in her body. Many start in the neck, head, scalp, and ears. Some report starting in the breasts and others "all over." The origin of the hot flash is not necessarily consistent for all women.

- The degree and amount of spread of the hot flash is also an individual thing; some spread up, some down, some in both directions, and some all over the body.
- Hot flashes occur for some women during the night. When they occur during the night they are called night sweats. Night sweats can be accompanied by profuse sweating and can interfere with sleep.
- The hot flash lasts from one-half to six minutes, although Dr. Perlmutter indicated that some can last for over 30 minutes.
- Hot flashes can occur over a number of years. Some women report having hot flashes for from five to ten years. If the hot flashes last over years, with time they decrease in intensity and frequency.
- Hot flashes vary in intensity from mild to moderate to severe.

Dr. Voda has described the three classifications as follows:

– *Mild* – barely noticeable, a feeling of warmth associated with either little or no perspiration; usually lasts for less than one minute and comes and goes without interfering with one's activities; sometimes accompanied by slight flushing; may include sensations of tingling and rushing blood.

– *Moderate* – warmer than mild; definitely noticeable; producing obvious visible perspiration in certain areas of the body; lasts two to three minutes; may include tingling, throbbing, rushing blood, light-headedness, chills, swelling of extremities, and a need to urinate; little interruption of normal activity.

– *Severe* – intensely hot; often causes woman to stop what she is doing and seek a cooling device; profound perspiration often over the entire body; lasts longer than the mild or moderate; causes more distraction and distressed feelings of not being able to cope may include waves of heat, dizziness, chills, suffocation, inability to concentrate, and chest pains.

- The same person, at different times, may experience different types of hot flashes.
- Ann Voda has conducted many studies into hot flashes. Her findings suggest that hot flashes vary in a systematic pattern throughout the day. "Though some women's experiences may differ, our research shows hot flashes most frequently occur

between the hours of 6 and 8 a.m., followed by a cooling-down period during the day. Frequency increases during evening hours of 6 and 10 p.m., followed by another cooling-down until 6 a.m. However, don't be alarmed if you have hot flashes only at night or only during the day. For some women this is the pattern." Ann Voda also pointed out that over a three-year period, while the number of hot flashes declined, the pattern of the flashes during the day remained very similar.

- Cold sweats is another term for a condition that seems related to hot flashes. They are usually described as a cold wetness around the forehead and the head. Sometimes the woman's hair gets wet or damp. Cold sweats have a slower buildup than hot flashes.

- Rosetta Reitz says, "The first thing to know about hot flashes is that they are harmless." She also says that they pass quickly and are nothing to be afraid of. Excellent advice.

Many attempts have been made to describe the types of things that may affect or trigger hot flashes. Again, it is necessary to remember that each person is an individual and the trigger for a hot flash for one person may not affect another the same way and that hot flashes can occur for no apparent reason. With this in mind, the following are a series of possible factors that may affect your hot flashes, if you have them:

- *Time of day* — The work of researchers such as Ann Voda has demonstrated consistent changes in the frequency of hot flashes over a period of a day.

- *Age* — As the menopausal woman becomes older, hot flashes decrease in frequency and intensity. Dr. Perlmutter noted that hot flashes can occur prior to the last menstrual period. The onset may be gradual and sporadic and may go unnoticed for several months or years. As menopause approaches, the woman feels the flashes become more frequent and more intense. A decline in the flashes occurs during the postmeno-pausal phase. Don't be surprised, however, if you hear of a woman in her seventies or eighties who has an occasional hot flash. It is minor in intensity and is very infrequent. There is no typical pattern that describes every woman.

- *Diet* — For some women, eating hot or spicy foods can affect their hot flashes. As I'll point out later, it is wise to watch your diet during this time.

- *Surgical removal of the ovaries* — When the ovaries are removed surgically (called an oophorectomy), some women can experience hot flashes soon after surgery. Some researchers feel that the probability of having hot flashes is greater after an oophorectomy than during natural menopause.
- *Stress, anxiety, excitement* — Some women reported that stress triggers their hot flashes.
- *Ambient temperature* — There is some discussion over the effect of temperature on hot flashes. Some report the same frequency of hot flashes during both warm and cold temperatures. Others feel there is a relationship between the day-to-day variation in the number of hot flashes and the ambient temperature. Ann Voda found that while there was no strong relationship between temperature and frequency of hot flashes, the duration of the flash was affected by the temperature.

Some of the questions women asked about hot flashes were as follows:

Can I know if I am a likely person to have hot flashes?
While considerable research is needed before hot flashes can be thoroughly understood, some researchers have been interested in speculating on an answer to this question. Ann Voda, for example, suggested that it may be that women who are most apt to develop hot flashes in menopause may be the ones who have a predisposition for either thermoregulatory problems or vascular instability, such as premenstrual headaches, migraines, or both. She also reported four women who, while still menstruating, described "nocturnal hyperthermia" where they were awakened at night with intense heat radiating from their bodies. She interpreted this finding as possibly indicating that the hot flash of menopausal women may be preceded by cyclic episodes of hyperthermia (i.e., high body temperatures) prior to the end of their menstrual periods.

Is there any way of knowing how long I will have hot flashes?
While it is difficult to give a general answer to this question, women can become familiar with their own pattern of the frequency, intensity, and duration of their hot flashes. If they do keep track of their own patterns, they will be able to see for themselves when the hot flashes are starting to decline.
When researchers are studying the pattern of hot flashes in

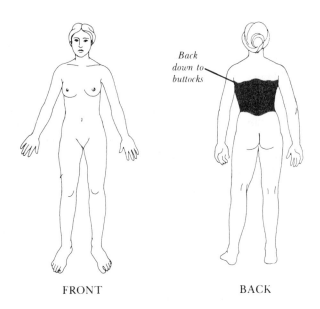

FRONT   **BACK**

SAMPLE HOT FLASH BODY DIAGRAM-ORIGIN

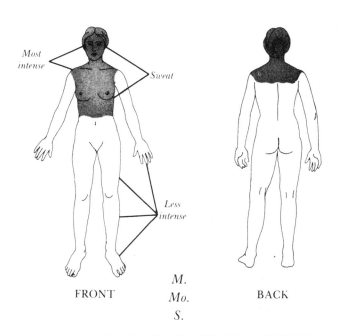

FRONT   **BACK**

SAMPLE HOT FLASH BODY DIAGRAM-SPREAD

women, they use body charts to indicate the point of origin and spread. I have included examples of body charts from Ann Voda's book. In it you can seen the areas involved in the hot flash, as well as how body charts are marked.

An alternative to the body chart is a diary or a chart where you can keep track of the origin, spread, frequency, duration, time of day, and, if you like, even what seemed to trigger the hot flash. As you can see on the hot flash Voda uses a code for the intensity of the flash: *M* for mild, *Mo* for moderate and *S* for severe.

You can keep track of whatever aspect of the hot flash seems to vary the most for you. For example, if the pattern of your hot flashes seems to vary little, it may be more important to jot down the duration or intensity, if they change.

The more information you have about your hot flashes the better you will understand your own pattern and any changes that occur. You may even discover things that you can do to avoid or reduce the number of hot flashes. Also, the more informed you are about yourself, the more concrete information you can give to your physician to help her/him prescribe an appropriate treatment for you.

What is the difference between a hot flash and a hot flush?
These two terms are confusing. Some writers do talk about hot flashes and flushes as being synonymous. Others differentiate between the hot flash, which is the subjective experience of warmth, and the hot flush, which is an observable change in colour, from pink to red.

What causes hot flashes ?
While there have been many studies designed to examine the cause of hot flashes, there is still more to learn. In the past, some felt that there was a psychological cause for them, without any physical basis. Researchers today seem to accept that hot flashes are related to lower levels of estrogen. For example, if there is a drop in estrogen, as there is following the surgical removal of the ovaries, hot flashes are more likely to occur. However, according to Dr. William Bates, a precondition for hot flashes seems to be estrogen exposure prior to withdrawal, since prepubertal girls or girls who do not go through menarche due to physical problems do not have hot flashes. Also, treatments which increase the

estrogen levels, as in estrogen replacement therapy, help the hot flash symptoms. However, this does not mean that there is a simple explanation relating to estrogen levels. Many studies have found that lutenizing hormone secretion accompanies hot flashes. For example, Dr. Tataryn and his colleagues measured plasma follicle stimulating hormone and lutenizing hormone around the time of the hot flash. They found that preceding each flash there was a release of pulsating lutenizing hormone but not of follicle stimulating hormone. The flash coincided with a fall in the plasma lutenizing hormone. But again, not every lutenizing hormone pulse is accompanied by hot flashes.

Drs. Casper and Yen, in a recent article on hot flashes, suggested that hot flashes represent what they call "dysfunctional thermoregulation initiated centrally in the hypothalamic thermoregulatory nuclei." In other words, a hot flash is a sign that the heat regulating system of the body is not functioning properly and that it is the hypothalamus (the part of the brain that is involved in menstruation) that controls this activity. They felt that peripheral dilation of the blood vessels that occurs during a hot flash with profuse perspiration are potent and characteristic component of heat loss mechanisms. They also suggested that the release of hypothalamic hormone, the gonadotropic releasing hormone which initiates the pituitary lutenizing hormone pulses, may be more directly related with the problems of thermoregulation during flashes. In turn the hypothalamus may be affected by more central areas of the brain.

How can I cope with hot flashes?

There have been many suggestions about how to cope with hot flashes. Drs. Casper and Yen reported a study in which the subjective (the woman's perception of the flash) and the objective (the physical measures taken when a flash occurs) flushes stopped immediately when the women went into a cold room. In a book titled, *Women Supporting Each Other*, it is suggested that a complete yoga breath, (a deep abdominal breath) when the hot flash begins is helpful. They also recommended cold temperatures and cotton clothing. Dr. Molnar advised applying cold cloths to the cheeks instead of the forehead or chest.

The most complete list of ideas of how to cope with a hot flash was in Ann Voda's booklet, *Menopause: Me and You.* She has eleven recommendations, which are summarized here:

1. "Don't worry, the hot flash is not a disease. It is a normal and natural part of menopausal experience. . . . Worrying about it may increase hot flash incidents.
2. "Know thyself. Keep a record or a diary of your hot flash. Time it, identify where it starts on your body and where it spreads. Try to identify your trigger(s), then work out ways of avoidance. . . . Others, though, report that daily record keeping forced them to pay more attention to their hot flash, made them think about it more, and made them miserable. Try it and see how it works for you. . . .
3. "Dress in the layered look. Many women cope with the heat sensation by taking off a layer or layers of clothing and then putting them back on as cooling commences. Others have found that certain fabrics are hot flash triggers: polyesters, for example, are avoided while cottons are preferred.
4. "Avoid hot areas. They trigger hot flashes for some women. Keep your thermostat at 65°, lower if possible. If you can't control the heat, dress in the layered look and keep a fan handy.
5. "Avoid highly seasoned, spicy foods, coffee, tea, and alcohol. These are common triggers for hot flashes. Try to find your specific trigger, but don't worry if you can't identify one. For some women a particular time of day is the trigger, suggesting that internally-triggered hot flashes are related to a resetting of biological rhythms.
6. "Avoid getting excited. Keep cool. . . if you can. Emotional stress is a trigger for some women.
7. "Stop the hot flash in its tracks! One woman stops flashes by imagining herself doing something very pleasurable. Another woman imagines herself walking in the snow without shoes, forcing herself to shiver, or anything to fool her body into being cool instead of hot. Other women cope quite well by seeking a cooling device: a fan, showering or applying cold cloths or ice cubes to certain body parts."
8. "Do not take tranquilizers or mood elevators. Psychotropic drugs are worthless against the hot flash.
9. "Consider vitamin therapy, but only after consulting a nurse, physician or nutritionist. Many women appear to relieve debilitating hot flashes with 400 I.U. of vitamin E and protein powder, yet others with vitamin C, 500 mg per day. For most women who use vitamins, research indicates that the hot flash is only relieved, not eliminated, and the relief is short-term.

10. "Be informed. There are possibly as many risks related to vitamin and over-the counter replacement substitutes as there are with estrogen use. Obtain as much reliable information as you can on health food replacements and on estrogen. The final word isn't in yet on what nutritional changes occur as we age. Nor do we know the long-term effects of estrogen use.

11. "Discuss your hot flashes with other women. Don't be a closet flasher. Most women are destined to experience hot flashes. The more you talk about it, the more natural it will become for women. The hot flash appears to be part of normal growth and development for women. Don't be ashamed of it."

What all of these suggestions have in common is that they stress the need for self-awareness and for knowledge about your body and the various things in your environment that affect you.

Osteoporosis

Osteoporosis is a disease in which there is an acceleration of the natural loss of bone mass to the point where it is below that expected when considering the person's age and sex. Associated with the loss in bone mass is an increased fragility in the bones. The skeleton may become so porous and brittle that the possibility of fractures is increased.

The probability of developing this disease increases for women after menopause. In the 1940s researchers proposed that osteoporosis was related to a loss of ovarian function and, therefore, decreased estrogen levels which were superimposed on age.

While the statistics vary slightly, it is usually reported that about one out of every four women will develop osteoporosis. This, however, is a topic where it is very difficult to collect accurate statistics, since some women may have the disease yet not show any symptoms. The primary symptom of osteoporosis is a susceptibility to bone fractures, particularly in the hip, wrist, and spine. These types of fractures seem to increase when women are over the age of 50 years. Spinal vertebrae may become so weak they collapse together in what is called a crush fracture. Women with this condition can become increasingly stooped, lose height, and can develop what is known as a Dowager's Hump. The drawings below will give you an idea of the apparent changes in the spine that occur with age.

FIGURE 2. Dowager's Hump

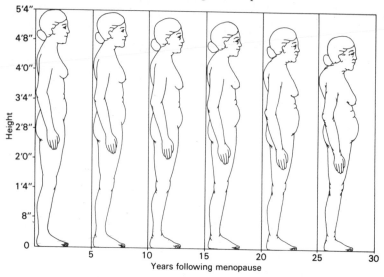

In order to understand what happens with osteoporosis. I would like to describe some information about bone formation. A very informative book call *Osteoporosis: How to Prevent the Brittle Bone Disease*, by Wendy Smith in consultation with Dr. Stanton Cohn, contains a very clear description. There are two principal forms of bone:

> "Trabecular bone is the spongy, metabolically active inner matter that comprises about twenty percent of the total skeleton; the remaining 80 percent is cortical (also called compact) bone — the thinner, smoother external envelope. Blood vessels and nerves flow through the bone tissue, which is impregnated with minerals, especially calcium and phosphorus. The proportions of the two types of bone vary greatly in different parts of the skeleton; their roles of age-related disease, susceptibility to fracture and response to treatment also differ widely." Throughout life, "both types of bone are continually remodeling: removing minerals from the bone tissue and releasing them into the blood and building up new tissue (formation). Until age eighteen or so, bones grow because formation exceeds resorption. After that, although bones are no longer growing in size, the body is still adding to their density . . . before the skeleton reaches its peak bone mas at approximately age 35 (even later for trabecular bone)."

Wendy Smith and Stanton Cohn describe two types of osteoporosis. They defined Type I as occurring six times more often in women, usually between the ages of 55 and 75 years. Trabecular bone loss is much greater than cortical and the fractures usually occur in the spinal vertebrae (the classic crush fracture) or the wrist. Type II osteoporosis is twice as frequent in women and is a disease of older people between the ages of 70 and 85 years. Trabecular and cortical bone are lost in equal amounts and the most common fracture sites are the hips and other long bones. Vertebrae fractures occur with less frequency.

How will I know if I have osteoporosis?
Researchers have stressed that it is sometimes difficult for women to identify that they have osteoporosis. One indicator, of course, is a decline in height. Also, lower back pain that does not radiate is another early symptom, although this could be caused by many other factors as well. As mentioned earlier, this disease is primarily without external symptoms. Fractures are often the basis for identification, especially when the intensity of the fall would not ordinarily have caused a break.

Wendy Smith and Stanton Cohn described another symptom you could look for to determine if you may have a problem with osteoporosis. They say that other areas to watch are your teeth and jaw. Although not a common occurrence, osteoporosis can cause periodontal problems. While there could be many causes for your teeth to become loose, it would be wise to check with your physician to see if this is an early sign of osteoporosis. Remember, the earlier you detect osteoporosis, the faster you can start to treat the symptoms.

How will my physician know if I have osteoporosis?
If you are high risk for osteoporosis, have some of the symptoms that may be related to the disease, or just are concerned, you would be wise to consult your physician. Physicians have several ways of measuring your bones. They have some techniques that can be used to gauge the bone mineral content. For example, the computerized axial tomography (CAT scan) measures the inner portion of the spinal vertebrae. Bear in mind that each of the techniques have their own side effects. Therefore, discuss each technique with your doctor and learn about what side effects may be involved before making your decision.

Conventional x-rays can detect bone loss but, according to some researchers, only when the loss is about 30 to 40 percent. Any of these methods can tell you about bone loss but cannot necessarily discover the women who are likely to sustain fractures. More indirect measures of assessing bone turnover include studies of calcium balance.

Are some women more prone to osteoporosis than others?
There is considerable evidence to show that some women are more prone to osteroporosis. Here are some of the risk factors:

- *Age*: As we get older there is an increased risk of osteoporosis. This is because of the change in our body chemistry. For example, the ability to absorb calcium effectively is diminished and our bodies need more vitamin D with age.
- *Sex*: Women are more prone than men to osteoporosis. Possibly due to the greater and earlier fluctuation in sex hormones, women begin to lose bone mass earlier than men. A simplistic explanation of this finding would be that the more bone mass you have, the more you have to lose before you become high risk for fractures. Also, men, generally, have greater peak bone mass. Some suggest that the sex differences are no longer present by the age of 80 years.
- *Menstrual problems*: Some researchers suggest that women who suffer from long term amenorrhea (the stopping of menstrual periods) prior to menopause are at greater risk. Also, women who experience menopause earlier are more prone to this disease.
- *Family history*: Some evidence indicates that there may be an as yet undetected genetic basis for a greater risk of osteoporosis. Possibly one factor that may explain this relationship is the possibility that peak bone mass may be genetically determined.
- *Size*: Women who are of small stature and have less bone mass are more at risk. As well, thin women are more likely to have problems than fat women. It has been suggested that the greater weight may stimulate the formation of more bone because of an increased load. Also, many feel that in post-menopausal women, fat tissue is one source of estrogen, since it is felt that the fatty tissues metabolize androgen into estrogen.
- *Skin color*: Women who are fair are at greater risk. Also, black women are less likely to contract osteoroporosis than white women.
- *Society*: Women in industrialized societies seem more prone to osteoporosis, perhaps due to their diet.

- *Exercise*: Women who exercise less are more likely to develop osteoporosis. One interpretation of this finding is that there is a direct relationship between exercise and the development of bone mass.
- *Alcohol use*: There is an increased risk of this disease in women who drink alcohol. It has been suggested that there is a decreased absorption of calcium and a negative effect on the integrity of the bone with alcohol use.
- *Smoking*: It has been reported that there is an increased likelihood of developing osteoporosis by women who smoke. A suggested interpretation is that there is less circulating estrogen and nicotine constricts the blood vessels and may impair nourishment of the bone.
- *Caffeine*: Caffeine has also been linked to an increased wastage of calcium. It may be that drinking a lot of coffee increases that proportion of calcium excreted in the urine and, therefore, less is being absorbed into the bones.
- *Magnesium deficiency*: Although there is some disagreement among experts, some believe that a magnesium deficiency will result in abnormal bone formation but the link with osteoporosis has not been established.
- *Antacids*: Aluminum contained in antacids has been found to hamper calcium absorption. It is important to read the contents carefully when taking antacids and choose one without aluminum.
- *Diet*: Many of us eat too much protein. Too much protein can cause an excess loss of calcium from the body.
- *Phosphorus*: The relationship between phosphorus intake and osteoporosis is a controversial issue. Some researchers feel that too much phosphorus interferes with calcium absorption. Others are less impressed with this factor as affecting the risk level of a woman
- *Fat absorption*: Again, this is a topic where evidence is not conclusive. However, some scientists feel that small amounts of fat enhance calcium absorption and large amounts impair it.
- *Oxalic acid*: Some foods contain an oxalic acid which has been reported by some researchers as having an adverse effect on calcium absorption. Such foods as spinach, parsley, and beet greens are high in both oxalic acid and calcium.
- *Drugs*: Some drugs, such as corticosteroids, used to treat arthritis, seem to cause bone loss when used over a prolonged period of time.

- *Low calcium diets*: Many women as they age do not maintain a diet that is high in calcium. Calcium has been reported to be an important mineral in remodeling bones. Calcium is present in many foods including dairy products.
- *Long-term immobilization*: Since physical exercise maintains general bone mass, long periods of bed rest can lead to bone loss.

Is there any way I can prevent osteoporosis?
There are many things that can be done to prevent or control osteoporosis:

- Be aware of the risk factors and avoid as many of them as possible.
- Good nutrition in childhood, when the bone mass is being developed, is important.
- Watch your diet and try to eat foods high in calcium and vitamin D and low in protein. (Keep in mind that too much vitamin D can become toxic.)
- Vigorous and continued exercise will help maintain bone mass. Regular exercise while the skeleton is growing will help to maximize peak bone mass in later life.

Can osteoporosis be treated and, if so, how?
Yes, there are many ways in which osteoporosis can be treated. One of the first things to be aware of is that it is important not to panic if you are diagnosed as having this disease. For some women it will affect their lives very little.

Wendy Smith and Stanton Cohn have summarized the available treatments for osteoporosis. These include:

- *Calcium supplementation*: Smith and Cohn consider this the first and most obvious step to take in treating osteoporosis.
- *Estrogen replacement therapy*: Evidence suggests that low doses of estrogen, as low as .3 mg per day, are adequate to halt bone loss, whereas, with higher doses, the likelihood of complications is increased. Care should be taken in determining whether you are a good candidate for estrogen replacement therapy and if you are, you should be closely monitored while taking it.
- *Exercise*: Moderate exercise is very good for people who have osteoporosis since it can slow down bone loss and even stimulate bone formation. Walking for 20 minutes three times a week, arm crossing, sideward bends, exercises to strengthen the

lower back and abdominal muscles are recommended. When planning an exercise program for yourself it is good to set it up with your physician or an expert in the field. Also, you have to keep in mind your general state of health and whether you have any other physical condition that may limit what kind of exercise you can do. Smith and Cohn recommend the following exercises for older women, although they would also be good exercises to do to help prevent the disease: brisk walking, stationary bicycling, calisthenics, jogging on a trampoline, ping-pong, rowing (on machines), square dancing, swimming, and water calisthenics.

- *Rest*: Proper rest is very important for relief from the pain of osteoporosis. The back strain can be relieved by periods of horizontal rest. "Try to manage without a pillow under your head; it will do more good under your knees to relieve strain on the back. Your bed should have a firm mattress too; proper support is all-important."

- *Experimental treatments* — A number of therapies that are in the experimental stage but that may increase bone mass include:

Parathyroid hormone — Low doses of a synthetic fragment of the parathyroid hormone seem to stimulate bone formation and increase the volume of trabecular bone in particular.

Oral phosphate — The administration of oral phosphate may also increase bone turnover by stimulating parathyroid hormone secretion.

ADFR — Smith and Cohn describe ADFR as an "as-yet-untested" theory of treatment. "It involves pulsing various agents into the body that will first activate bone remodeling, then depress the resorption phase, then leave a free period for uninhibited bone formation, then repeat the entire cycle."

Hormonal vitamin D3 — Since there is evidence that in osteoporosis there is no proper metabolizing of Vitamin D into its active form, which affects the absorption of calcium, Calcitriol (the name for this hormonal form) should improve calcium absorption.

PEMF — This treatment is also experimental and not yet widely used. With Pulsed Electromagnetic Fields, a "specially fitted electrical device is placed over the broken bone; the pulsed field it produces is believed to help bones heal more rapidly."

Sodium fluoride — Sodium fluoride has been used as a treatment, sometimes in combination with calcium. There are, however, some problems with this treatment, since there are side effects associated with it, such as gastric irritation, nausea, ulcers, pains in the legs, ankles or feet.

Osteoporosis is a condition that can affect one in every four women. It is important, therefore, for each of us who is either pre-, peri-or postmenopausal to understand the symptoms, risk factors, and treatment available. An understanding of this disease can, in some cases, help us to avoid some of the risk factors and to cope with the symptoms if and when they occur. An additional factor to be aware of is that in some of the major cities there is an Osteoporosis Society that is set up to provide women with support and knowledge. This type of support can be very informative and helpful. Also, some of the major hospitals offer exercise programmes that are specifically designed for women who have osteoporosis. Again, this type of setting would provide an opportunity to discuss with other women their way of dealing with the problems they encounter.

Just how universal are menopausal symptoms ?

While I have described for you a series of symptoms that are related to menopause in Western societies, it is clear that women differ considerably in their individual types, patterns, frquency, and duration of symptoms and in their ability to cope with them. Several anthropologists have examined menopause in different countries in an attempt to clarify symptoms and the factors that affect them. Cross-cultural research has helped our understanding of several issues relating to menopausal symptoms. Anthropologists have interviewed or observed women to understand which symptoms occur in different cultures, whether there are differences in the age of menopause, the different attitudes of societies to menopause, and whether these attitudes seem to affect the occurrence of symptoms. Studies have been carried out in many different countries, including Japan, Mexico, Greece, Indonesia, Israel, and in Europe.

In general, cross-cultural studies reinforce the conclusion that the understanding of menopausal symptoms is very complex.

Firstly, within each culture are different myths and information which result in a description of menopause as a physiological or psychosocial event and define the expected characteristics of perimenopausal women. These expectations and stereotypes are available to not only the women in the culture but also their husbands, children, co-workers, physicians, and other members of the community. Dr. Kaufert felt that these expectations formed a filter through which the physiological sensations arising from fluctuating hormonal levels were experienced. She found that in some cultures the stereotypes were positive and in others negative.

It has also been shown that women may be given different roles within their society depending on their menopausal status. In some cultures, women are rejected when they can no longer produce children. In others, as they become menopausal, women's status improves. They are allowed to do several things that were previously taboo for them. For example, some societies allow women to become involved in what were previously considered "male" activities, such as drinking, being involved in important societal ceremonies, and becoming a shaman or medicine man, all of which are considered to be of value in the society.

Joel Wilbush, in 1985 indicated another interesting explanation of why different symptoms are reported in different cultures. He explained the variations between cultures by indicating that the social and cultural background influenced the women's interpretation of symptoms. He commented that subliminal sensations, ignored in one culture, are accepted as symptoms in another. In other words, the subjective sensations which are ignored in many cultures are the symptoms of menopause as experienced by Western women. He felt that women of all cultures are aware of similar sensations.

Another interpretation of menopausal symptoms is from the research of Patricia Kaufert. Based on her review of the literature, she felt that a woman whose existing level of self-esteem is high will be less vulnerable to a negative stereotype than a woman whose self-esteem is low. She commented that several factors can affect self-esteem, including the presence or absence of confiding relationships. It is interesting to note that social support has been found to affect attitudes to various life events, such as pregnancy. The levels of self-esteem would also depend on the values within different cultures. Kaufert also felt that hormone levels may be influenced by psychological variables; possibly they fluctuate more widely with women whose self-esteem makes them more vulnerable to stress caused by a negative stereotype of menopause.

When looking at how women experience menopause in different cultures, it becomes clear just how complex the variation of symptoms is. For example, Margaret Lock reported in 1986 some preliminary results of her research in Japan. She compared the menopausal symptoms of a group of women from a city, farm, and factory. She found that menopause in Japan was considered an event of no great importance; it was viewed as a life cycle transition and as a natural part of the aging process. In addition, even the language used to describe menopausal symptoms was different. For example, there was no word for hot flashes. The symptoms most frequently reported by the Japanese women were headaches, shoulder stiffness, lumbago, irritability, loss of energy, tiredness and general debility, weakening eyesight, and gray hair. All of these symptoms seem more related to aging than menopause. In a study conducted in Manitoba, Canada, by Patricia Kaufert, peri- and postmenopausal women reported experiencing hot flashes (12.6 and 10.8 percent respectively), while 14.9 percent of premenopausal women indicated the same thing.

That some women from certain cultures do not describe the "typical" Western symptoms of menopause was also apparent in the research by Marcha Flint. She studied a group of women from Northern India, where women emerge from a more restricted role and become freer in their behaviour when they become menopausal. In this group she found a symptom-free perimenopausal period.

The effect of culture on women's reactions to menopause can be seen in the research by Yewoubda Beyene with Mayan and Greek women. Both groups of women were from traditional villages. While the women seemed to share similar cultural values with respect to beliefs and practices regarding menstruation, child rearing and their other roles, they experienced differences during menopause. In both cultures the roles of good mother, housekeeper, and hard worker were valued. Old age is associated with increased power and respect, particularly for married women. Menopause is not considered a life crisis nor a psychological nor physiological problem. The only recognized symptom is irregularity and final cessation of menstruation. In the Greek village, menopause was associated with growing old, not having energy, and a general downhill life course. In this group, 73 percent had hot flashes, 30 percent cold sweats, 42 percent headaches and dizziness, 30 percent insomnia, 12 percent hemorrhage.

These symptoms were regarded as natural and causing only temporary discomfort.

From her research Dr. Beyene concluded that the perception and experience of menopause varies cross-culturally and that this difference is not simply explained by role changes or cultural taboos. She suggested that diet, fertility, and genetic background may help to explain the differences.

Dona Lee Davis, an anthropologist, also examined the relationship between culture and menopause in a fishing village in Newfoundland in Canada. Emphasis in this culture was more on age than on menstrual pattern. Change was considered a normal part of aging. The most common symptom reported by middle-aged women was "nerves." They felt that nerves aged at a greater rate than other body structures.

There are many other studies in different parts of the world that show varied patterns of symptoms to menopause depending on the cultural context. There are, however, a few studies that tend to support more a biological interpretation of menopause. Anthropologist Ann Wright compared traditional and acculturated Navajo women. They differed in whether or not they were educated, spoke English, and the type of work they did, for example whether or not it was outside the home. She found that the prevalence of symptoms was very similar for both groups of Navajo and European women. Hot flashes were the most frequent symptoms. However, the pattern of symptoms was different; the Navajo reported hot flashes occurred less frequently.

Cross-cultural studies have also been of value in looking at the age at which menopause occurs. In only a few of the studies did there seem to be any difference from Western women. Dr. Walker and his colleagues found that black women in three rural and urban areas in South African started menopause at the same age as North American women, that is around 49 or 50 years. However, the Mayan women in Beyene's research experienced menopause at an average age of 42 years.

The experience of menopause depends of a complex interaction of many factors. While we do not know exactly how each factor in the culture interacts with hormonal changes to result in each woman's individual experience of menopause, we do know that some characteristics may make women more vulnerable to certain types of symptoms.

What this means is that there may be some similarity in the age of menopause and types of symptoms with your mother, if genetic factors are, in fact, important. However, if you are perimenopausal, you cannot predict what your symptoms or manner of dealing with them will be, because of the complex number of factors that interact to produce your reactions.

The complexity of the issues involved in a woman's reactions means that you do not have a clear behaviour pattern you can expect from a perimenopausal woman, and no one should expect them from you. If a perimenopausal woman is depressed or irritable there may be reason other than the simple fact of menopause. If it is your friend or relative, check with her to see what is causing her actions. If other people are making assumptions about you, you would be wise to correct them when they are wrong.

As Margaret Lock commented in 1986, "The best executed studies reveal that simple associations between such variables as 'empty nest' and a high incidence of menopausal symptoms, or release from female role restrictions and low incidence of menopausal symptoms, are not generalizable either within or between populations."

Chapter Five

Treatment of Menopausal Symptoms

Drug therapy
Many women hear conflicting stories of the way they can be relieved of their menopausal symptoms. One of the most controversial topics is whether drugs are the most appropriate form of treatment. Hormone replacement therapy, tranquilizers, antidepressants, and sleeping pills are some of the drugs prescribed for the menopausal woman. Of these, hormone replacement therapy has been the most researched and discussed and is the most confusing.

Estrogen therapy has been used to treat menopausal symptoms since the 1920s. In the 1960s, Dr. Robert Wilson, in his book *Feminine Forever*, pronounced that the "following clinical facts are now firmly established."

"Menopause is curable. Under proper treatment, nearly all symptoms cease in the vast majority of cases. The bodily changes typical of middle age can be reversed, and sexual functions can be restored, along with a fully feminine appearance. The only sexual function that cannot be restored is fertility.

"Menopause is completely preventable. No woman need suffer menopause or any of its symptoms if she receives preventive treatment before the onset of menopause."

Dr. Wilson, in his book and articles in popular magazines, told women that estrogen replacment therapy was a cure for their estrogen-deficiency disease. Estrogen was the youth pill that would keep them feminine forever. "Every woman alive today has the option of remaining feminine forever," he wrote. Many women were influenced by Dr. Wilson's writings and estrogen became the preferred treatment for many menopausal women. According to Barbara and Gideon Seaman, by the 1970s, Premarin, a form of estrogen, had become the fourth or fifth most popular drug in the United States. However, by the '70s, researchers began to be concerned about the relationship between endometrial cancer (cancer of the lining of the uterus) and estrogen replacement therapy (ERT). By this time it was also known that Dr. Wilson's research had been financed by one of the drug companies that sold estrogen pills, which affected his credibility. Other evidence started to link ERT to a number of side effects, such as breast cancer, gall bladder disease, and uterine bleeding. By the mid '70s, drug companies in the United States were required to list the possible side effects in their advertising for ERT. As the women's movement developed, many writers began promoting the right of women to make their own decisions about treatment for their symptoms. They were also suggesting that women consider the use of more natural forms of treatment, such as diet, vitamin supplements, and exercise. There is now a considerable body of research on ERT but a great deal of disagreement about its benefits and risks remains:

- "My doctor advised me to take estrogen within five years and if my G.P. would not give it to me, he would. I have concerns about the safety of it but I didn't mention it because I'll probably look for a different gynecologist."
- "My physician recommended hormones. I disagreed with this."
- "My doctor said he wanted to give me some hormone therapy and I told him I wanted to do without it for the time being and see how I felt."
- "My doctor told me to take estrogen but I was concerned about what I had read about the side effects and I did not want to take a chance."

On the other hand, estrogen therapy has helped some women:

- "I'm taking medication and it has been very successful."
- "I was determined to get through my menopause on my own but I had problems with hot flashes and found that estrogen helped me."
- "Estrogen helped me get through a very difficult time."

From the available research, it is clear that estrogen can be beneficial in certain cases. However, women differ in their therapeutic needs. It is important to thoroughly investigate the risks and benefits for yourself before making a decision about whether to use ERT.

How do I know if estrogen replacement therapy is for me?

Menopausal women differ in their symptoms, tolerance for symptoms, additional stressors in their lives, and therapeutic preferences. If you are considering the use of ERT, you should familiarize yourself with the possible benefits, risks and contraindications.

Benefits of ERT

The research on the benefits of ERT is by no means consistent. However, several studies have suggested that for some women ERT can be beneficial for:

- *The relief of hot flashes* — ERT has been shown to reduce the frequency and severity of hot flashes more effectively than other forms of treatment such as vitamin E, sedatives, and clonidine (an anit-hypertensial drug). For some women the hot flashes may resume after cessation of the ERT. Keep in mind, however, that hot flashes will subside on their own, usually within one to five years after the menopause.
- *Vaginal atrophy* — ERT can relieve the symptoms associated with the increasing dryness of the vagina that accompany menopause. Again, when the ERT is stopped, the symptoms will recur.
- *Osteoporosis* — ERT has been demonstrated to help prevent bone resorption associated with osteoporosis and bone fracture. However, it does not cure osteoporosis and the length of the protective effect is not known, although some research has suggested the effects may last from five to ten years. Women who are more likely to be at risk for osteoporosis, such as Caucasian women with small body frames and who smoke, are often given ERT as a preventative measure.
- *Cardiovascular disease* — While the research is inconclusive and some researchers have stated that the reduction of coronary heart disease cannot at the present time be considered a proven benefit of ERT, a number of studies have suggested that ERT can increase the levels of high-density lipoproteins and decrease the low density lipoproteins that are associated with lower levels

of cholesterol. The high density lipoproteins and lower cholesterol have been related to a decreased risk of atherosclerosis. In addition, estrogen has been found in some research to lower the risk of coronary heart disease in women who have had both ovaries removed (bilateral oophorectomy).

- *Feelings of well-being* — Many women seem to feel better, have an improved self image, and be less depressed when they are taking ERT. This effect may be secondary to relief from hot flashes and night sweats. It might also be related to the quality of sleep. Studies have demonstrated that women who were taking ERT increased the amount of rapid eye movement (REM) sleep, associated with a more peaceful sleep, and lessened the time required to fall asleep.
- *Memory* — Some women have found that their memory seems to be impaired during the climacteric and menopausal years. With ERT, some women experienced improved concentration and memory skills. "I find that when I stop taking my ERT, I have more problems with concentration and memory." It is very likely that what is affecting the memory is the reduction in hot flashes and night sweats.
- *Formication* — Formication, or the feeling of skin crawling, has been reported as being controlled by the use of ERT.
- *Surgical or natural menopause before the age of 40* — Premature menopause has been associated with more severe hot flashes and an increased risk of osteoporosis. Therefore, ERT is helpful in limiting menopausal symptoms for these women.

Some researchers have discussed the possibility that the benefits of ERT may be due to placebo effects. Studies have found that women given a placebo, that is a pill that has no pharmacological effects and is effective in treating a condition only because the person believes that it will, also report a decrease in the frequency and severity of their hot flashes. However, there are other studies that have failed to demonstrate similar placebo effects.

Risks of ERT
There has been a great deal of debate in the research literature about the risks that are associated with the use of ERT.

- *Endometrial cancer*— Many studies have demonstrated a relationship between ERT and endometrial cancer, or cancer of the lining of the uterus. The Third National Cancer Survey found that the annual incidence of endometrial cancer is 0.7/1000 women. The use of ERT increased the rate to 2.3 to 3.0/1000. Some researchers stress that while the risk of endometrial cancer is increased with ERT, the magnitude of the increase is low. Also, if the cancer is detected and treated early, the cure rate is high. The women who are at most risk for endometrial cancer are obese (because of the conversion of androgen in the fatty tissues to a form of estrogen); are taking high doses of ERT; and have been using ERT for a long period. Many studies have suggested that the addition of a progesterone (progestin) during the last seven to ten days of the estrogen therapy may prevent the development of this form of cancer.

- *Breast cancer* — The breast consists of tissues that are dependent on and responsive to estrogen. Some research has shown that exposure to estrogen, particularly in a low progesterone environment, is associated with the growth of breast tumors. It has been suggested that these tumors may be the result of an increased intake of estradiol (one form of estrogen) due to many factors affecting the serum binding rather than the total estrogen levels. The incidence of breast cancer is reported to be higher in those women who have experienced an early menarche or a late menopause and, therefore, who are exposed to longer periods of estrogen unopposed by progesterone. Women who have had an oophorectomy before menopause are at lower risk of breast cancer. The research on breast cancer is, however, less consistent and there are well-designed studies that have not shown an increase in breast cancer related to ERT. It is clear that some women are at greater risk for breast cancer, for example those who have a history of benign breast disease. These women should not take ERT. Some researchers feel that if there is a history of breast cancer in the family, ERT should be avoided.

- *Gall bladder disease* — There is an increase of problems with gall bladder stones in women who are using ERT. Clare Edman described the development of gall stones as being due to the bile becoming saturated with cholesterol during estrogen therapy and combining with other metabolic salts to form stones. Obese women who are taking ERT seem to be more at risk for gall stones. Again, this is probably because of the increased levels of estrogen in their bodies in the fatty tissue.

- *Depletion of vitamins* —It has been reported that women who have been using estrogens for a year may need to take vitamin supplements, particularly vitamin B6, since the hormone therapy seems to deplete the amount of B6 in the body. Since lower levels of B6 have been related to depression, some clinicians and researchers feel it is important to take a supplement.

- *Edema*— Fluid retention in the tissues has been a side effect for some women on ERT. It has been suggested that when this problem occurs, the woman is on too high a dosage of ERT and lowering the dosage should stop fluid retention.

- *Uterine bleeding* — Some research has suggested that a third of the women on estrogen will have some bleeding during the use of ERT. If this occurs, you should be carefully examined because of the relationship between ERT and endometrial cancer. Also, if you are taking a combination of estrogen and progesterone you will have regular menstrual bleeding. The amount of uterine bleeding also seems to be related to the amount of hormones taken.

- *Facial scars* — Barbara and Gideon Seaman described a condition called porophyria, which is "sometimes hereditary, and sometimes a reaction to drugs including estrogen. It may involve the excessive growth of facial hair, abnormalities of pigment metabolism, and large skin swellings that form scar tissue as they heal."

- *Other symptoms* such as breast tenderness, increased vaginal discharge, and leg cramps also have been found to be related to ERT.

In addition to the above, there are several other possible side effects that may occur when using ERT. For an example, I looked at the side effects listed for Premarin, a very commonly used form of ERT. The *Compendium of Pharmaceuticals and Specialties* describes the potential adverse reactions that have been reported by some women using estrogen. These include nausea, jaundice, increase or decrease in body weight, breakthrough bleeding, spotting and withdrawal bleeding, increased cervical mucus, endometrial hyperplasia, reactivation of endometriosis, sodium and salt retention, breast swelling and tenderness, increased blood sugar levels, decreased glucose tolerance, headaches, increase or decrease of libido, allergic reactions and rashes, an increase in blood pressure in susceptible people, and aggravation of migraine headaches. A relationship with thrombophlebitis, pulmonary embolism, and cerebral thrombosis and the use of oral contraceptive preparations containing estrogen has also been established in some studies. When reading this list keep in mind that these are only *possible* side effects, which means they are not necessarily experienced by all women on ERT. In fact, the research does suggest that a decrease in glucose tolerance, increase in thrombophlebitis, pulmonary embolism, and cerebral thrombosis are not consistently found with menopausal women taking ERT. It is important, however, to be as well informed as possible about any drug before taking it. Be aware of your own medical history and ask your doctor if you have any questions. Some women have said they felt a little reluctant about talking to their physicians about their concerns. It may help to think that even though it is unlikely that you will have a certain side effect, it is your own health that is at stake.

There are those who feel that an additional risk in using ERT for menopausal symptoms is that women can become psychologically dependent on the drug and that their ability to "get through the menopause" depends on the medication. There were some who wanted to experience their menopause naturally. This difference of opinion depends partly on how severe the symptoms are.

Contraindications with ERT
It would seem unwise to use ERT if you have any of the following problems: undiagnosed vaginal bleeding, liver or cerebrovascular disease, pulmonary embolism (blood clot), breast or uterine tumors, gall bladder disease, hypertension, past history of endometriosis, severe varicose veins, or severe obesity. Some clinicians and researchers also feel ERT may be contraindicated if you smoke heavily.

Whether or not you are going to take estrogen is an important issue. In making your decision, you may want to consider the following questions.

• What is your physician recommending and why?
• How are you feeling?
• Do you have menopausal symptoms, such as hot flashes, or problems with sexual intercourse?
• If you do have symptoms, have you tried other, more natural treatments, such as diet, vitamins, and exercise?
• Have you noticed a difference in your height?
• Do you still menstruate? If so, is your menstrual cycle regular? Is the flow changing? Is it excessive?
• Is there any problem in your medical history that might be complicated with ERT, such as high blood pressure or breast tumors?

- Are you having breakthrough bleeding after having stopped menstruating for a long period of time?
- Do you have a family history of early heart attacks, high cholesterol, high blood pressure, or breast tumors?
- Are there extra stresses in your life that are bothering you?
- How do you feel about taking medication?
- Would you describe yourself as overweight?
- Do you smoke? If so, how heavily?

Answering these questions may help you come to some decisions for yourself.

What is the difference between natural and synthetic estrogen?
Natural and synthetic estrogens are both used for menopausal symptoms. Natural estrogens, sometimes called conjugated estrogens, are those that are derived from animal sources. For example, Premarin is one of most popular natural estrogens. Premarin comes from the urine of pregnant mares. In fact, that is how it got its name: **Pregnant-mare's urine.** Synthetic estrogens are synthesized within the laboratory and are made to resemble natural estrogens. Diethylstilbestrol is a synthetic estrogen. They tend to cost less but seem to have more side effects, such as nausea. Some researchers have suggested that natural estrogens are better because they decrease the risk of cardiovascular problems. However, there are some researchers who have not found either a difference in side effects or in the lessened risk of blood clotting. To be safe, you would probably be wise to use a natural estrogen if you are undergoing ERT.

What kinds of hormone replacement are there?
Hormone pills are the most frequently used form of ERT. They differ in whether they are straight estrogen or are estrogen combined with other drugs. Estrogen has been combined with male hormones (testosterone), vitamins, and tranquilizers. Progesterone pills are also available. Different combinations are prescribed depending on the particular symptoms. For example, male hormones may be used where one of the symptoms is lack of sex drive or tranquilizers could be administered for anxiety. If you are taking a combination of drugs, it is important to know what you are taking and what the possible side effects of the additional drug may be.

One of the widely debated issues in hormone treatment at the moment is whether progesterone should be combined with estrogen. The use of such a combination is called hormone replacement therapy.

Progesterone is believed to help prevent endometrial cancer. Others believe it provides protection against breast cancer. Drs. Meeks and Bates, in a recent article, explained that progesterone modifies the effects of estrogen on target tissues by decreasing the number of estrogen receptors in those tissues and by inducing an enzyme that reduces the tissue concentration of estradiol (a more potent form of estrogen) to a less potent form, estrone.

HRT will cause vaginal bleeding on a regular basis. Susan Flamholtz Trien reported a study which stated that 97 percent of women will experience bleeding until age 60 and by age 65, only 60 percent still have bleeding. She also noted that the bleeding is usually shorter and scantier, lasting two or three days each month. Whether vaginal bleeding occurs may be dependent on the amount of progesterone used. In a recent study by A.L. Magos and colleagues, low levels of progesterone were taken daily in combination with the estrogen. They found it was possible to maintain the protective aspects of progesterone against endometrial cancer but without any bleeding. Obviously, progesterone is recommended more for women whose vaginas have not been surgically removed, although some physicians still prescribe progesterone even if they have been.

There is a considerable amount of research being carried out on progesterone. Many clinicians and researchers feel that the combination of estrogen and progesterone more closely matches the premenopausal cycle of hormones and is, therefore, more natural. However, a great deal needs to be learned about the proper dosages, timing, and long-term effects. In fact, some researchers still feel that there is no proof that progesterone counteracts the carcinogenic properties of estrogen. Drs. Meeks and Bates commented that the beneficial effects of estrogen on lipid profiles may be altered depending on which progesterone agent is employed.

Are there any advantages to taking pills or injections for hormone therapy?
There are several ways in which hormone replacement therapy can be given: orally in the form of a pill, by injection, topical creams, vaginal ring, wafers under the tongue or implants.

- *Pills* — The most usual way to take hormones is in pill form. When the pill is swallowed the hormones go through the stomach, intestines, and liver before entering the bloodstream. Therefore, by the time it gets into the bloodstream, it is less concentrated than when first taken. The usual method is to take estrogen for three weeks and nothing for one week. If progesterone is also part of your treatment, it is usually taken with the estrogen during the last seven to ten days of the "on" cycle. The main advantage of taking hormone replacement therapy in pill form is that if side effects occur the dosage can be changed easily. The disadvantages are that a woman has to remember to take her pills and it is a less efficient way of taking estrogen, since some of the drug is absorbed in the liver. Also, in the few cases where blood pressure was increased during HRT, it was when estrogen was taken orally. Drs. Winnifred Cutler, Celso-Ramón Garcia and David Edwards explain this as being due to the liver responding quickly to the oral ingestion of hormones. Increases in blood molecules that sometimes increase the risk of hypertension (high blood pressure) have been observed during orally administered HRT. These molecules do not increase when estrogen is taken in other ways.
- *Injections* — Injections of estrogen, or estrogen in combination with other drugs, last usually for about a month. The disadvantages of this method are that the woman has to get what may be a painful injection every month and side effects cannot be remedied until the effectiveness of the drug declines. Some researchers are concerned about the effects of the sudden surge of hormones experienced with an injection.
- *Topical creams* — Hormone creams applied directly to the skin are absorbed into the bloodstream. They can be applied when needed directly on the vulva and vagina. This method can be used both for the treatment of vaginal atrophy and for any other menopausal symptom. One advantage of using topical creams is that the liver is not affected. Since the cream is not diluted in the same way the pills are, less estrogen is necessary to control symptoms. The main disadvantage is the messiness of a vaginal cream. Some women find suppositories are more convenient.
- *Vaginal ring* — This method is in the experimental stage and more research needs to be done before it will be available for general use. The ring containing estrogen is placed in the vag-

ina where it releases the hormone at a constant rate. The ring is easy to insert and remove and may be left in place during intercourse.

- *Estrogen wafers* — These are placed under your tongue every other day. The wafer dissolves and is absorbed very quickly into the bloodstream. Since the wafer is swallowed it goes into the digestive track. Smaller amounts of estrogen go to the liver using this method than when a pill is taken. This method is not as effective in treating vaginal atrophy as the cream because lower levels of the drug reach the vaginal tissues.

- *Implants*— Implants have been used for the past 30 years in the United Kingdom and France. They are considered in the experimental stage in the United States and are not available in Canada. Implants were designed to achieve more continuous and uniform levels of hormones in the blood. Small pellets are implanted under local anaesthetic. A tiny incision is made in the hip or above the pubic area. The pellet is effective in controlling symptoms for periods of three to six months. By this time the pellet has been absorbed and another pellet has to be implanted. In some research the effects over a three-year period have been shown to reproduce the balance of the different estrogens better than the oral therapies. With this method estrogen can be used alone or in combination with other hormones. There has been some recent research that has examined the combination of estrogen, progesterone, and testosterone for the treatment of loss of sex drive. The implant of combined hormones was found to be effective in the treatment of both the sex drive and other menopausal symptoms. The advantages of this technique were described by Dr. Whitehead as follows: the rate of absorption is slower and continuous; the effective dosage of combined hormones is less than the dosage of each hormone taken separately; implants do not cause gastric or intestinal symptoms; the woman is not continually reminded of her condition by taking pills; and no thrombosis or embolism has been observed. The disadvantages are the expense; the need for minor surgery; and the necessity of removing the pellet if side effects do occur. The only alternative to removal is the woman suffering any problems over a long period of time. As with the other techniques, more research is necessary to understand more fully its effects.

How can I tell if the amount of hormones I am taking is right for me?

The basic principle behind the HRT is that you want to take the smallest amount necessary to control your menopausal symptoms. Your physician will recommend a dosage based on the method of administration (each method has a range of doses that are usually given), the type of symptoms you have, and other factors such as your age, menstrual history, and number of children. It is very important for you to monitor your own feelings and symptoms when you are taking hormone treatment. According to the recent research, relatively low doses of hormones can be effective in relieving your symptoms. Remember that the larger the dose of the hormones, the more likley you are to develop problems.

Why do doctors want me to take hormone treatment?

Many women have commented that their physicians have wanted them to take hormone replacement therapy and they were not interested. There are several reasons that physicians may encourage their patients to take HRT:

- Physicians tend to see menopausal women who have problems and who need help. They have seen many women benefit from taking HRT but they are not exposed to a general population of menopausal women, many of whom are successfully managing their menopause without treatment.
- They are constantly exposed to advertising in medical journals that represent the menopausal woman as someone suffering from an estrogen deficiency disease. For example, a sad, wrinkled woman with pursed lips is pictured over the words "You see her from 45 to 55 with hot flashes, night sweats, fatigue, headache, palpitations, emotional distress . . . treat her with Premarin . . . keep her on Premarin . . . replacement therapy at any stage." Or an older woman with a furrowed brow is sitting in a chair with a rather longing expression on her face and the words "Born too soon" are superimposed on the side of the picture. The copy reads "to have benefited from estrogen replacement therapy during her menopausal years — but even now, it is not too late to institute treatment for the postmenopausal syndrome." Or in another advertisement there are three "No's" in big letters. In the "o" of each no is a different picture. In the first one a man is looking rather rejected, supporting his head on his hand. In the second "o" is a

group of people all dressed up, and in the third "o" is a rather sad, lonely child. On the next page the copy reads: "When symptoms of the menopause make her say 'no' because of atrophic vaginitis; 'no' because of moderate to severe vasomotor symptoms [it is curtailing her social activities and making her stay home]; 'no' because of postmenopausal osteoporosis [she cannot play with her little granddaughter]."

• In a recent article, Gloria Cowan, Lynda Warren and Joyce Young measured the attitudes to menopausal symptoms and their treatment in a group of physicians, nurses, menopausal and postmenopausal women. The women emphasized somatic symptoms, such as hot flushes, while the physicians stressed the psychological ones. Physicians rated estrogen and counseling more favorably than either the women or nurses. The results suggested that the medical perception of menopause stressed symptom pathology and psychological causes more than the women did. As Dr. Sloane stated in 1980, physicians believe menopause to be more traumatic than most women.

• Also, physicians vary in their background training and experience with menopausal symptoms and women.

What happen if I have menopausal symptoms that require treatment and I can't take estrogen?

When women cannot take estrogen, the male hormones of androgen and testosterone are sometimes given for the relief of menopausal symptoms. However, they do not tend to be as effective as estrogen and can produce side effects such as deepening and lowering of the voice or the appearance of coarse facial hairs. There are also the more natural forms of treatment available, such as diet, vitamins, and exercise. For example, calcium supplements can treat or help prevent osteoporosis when estrogen cannot be taken.

Some general issues about hormone replacement therapy

• Make sure you are well informed about your symptoms and alternative forms of treatment before making a decision about HRT.

• Take an active role in the decision.

• If you are taking HRT, try to ensure you are taking the smallest dose for the shortest period of time, while maximizing your own comfort.

• Keep track of your own symptoms so you know how you are progressing.

• Have a very careful medical assessment done before starting treatment. According to Dr. McArthur, this should include a detailed medical history, complete physical and pelvic examination, careful recording of blood pressure, a baseline xeromammogram (a technique involving the use of x-rays or infrared photographs of the breast to check for the presence of growths), a papanicolaou smear (a Pap smear is a test in which a specimen of tissue is taken from the cervix or womb and examined under the microscope for the presence of abnormal cells), endometrial biopsy (an in-office procedure in which a small instrument is placed into the uterus and a sample of the endometrium is obtained. This sample is then used to analyze for the presence of abnormal cells. This procedure sometimes causes menstrual-type cramping during and after the experience.), and tests for fasting plasma glucose, cholesterol, and triglycerides (which gives an indication of the storage of fats in the body).

• Careful monitoring by both you and your physician are an important part of HRT. Your blood pressure should be checked and a pelvic and breast examination should be carried out every six months to a year. Also, many physicians recommend that an annual endometrial biopsy should be done. You can monitor your own symptoms by keeping track of their frequency, duration, and intensity. A regular breast self-examination is another essential part of your monitoring. Any breast examination involves three parts. First is a visual inspection in front of a mirror where you look for any changes in shape of your breasts, their colour or skin texture. This is done with your arms by your sides, behind your head and on your hips. Secondly probing your breasts in a circular motion from the outside to the inside, and thirdly gently squeezing the nipple. These last two steps should be done once while lying down and again in a sitting position. Place your right hand behind your head while you examine your right breast, the left while checking your left breast. Some women prefer to do the last examination while in the shower. You can use some skin cream, or the soap in your shower, to move your hands more freely. Use the pads of your fingers, not your fingertips. Checking your breasts regularly is an important part of caring for yourself. As you get to know your own body better, you will become aware of any changes. Breast examinations should become easier as you get older, since you are not going through cyclical hormonal changes which can affect them. You could check with your physician to make sure you are doing your self examination properly.

What are the other forms of medication used for the treatment of menopausal women ?
In addition to, or instead of, HRT there are other forms of medication that have been prescribed for menopausal women. Tranquilizers, anti-depressants, and sleeping pills are used to treat the symptoms of nervousness, anxiety, irritability, depression, insomnia, and fatigue. Also, when HRT cannot be used, tranquilizers or anti-depressants have been suggested as a treatment for hot flashes. Some physicians also prescribe a drug, clonidine, normally used for high blood pressure. These different drugs tend not to be as effective as HRT in controlling menopausal symptoms. In addition, each one has its own side effects, adverse drug effects, and possibilities for interacting with other types of medication. For example, the possible side effects of clonidine are dry mouth, drowsiness, constipation, dizziness, headache, and fatigue. One can also develop a tolerance to clonidine, so that the amount you take to achieve the same effect may increase over time. The possible adverse drug effects, while infrequent, include loss of appetite, nausea, vomiting, weight gain, breast enlargement, various effects on the heart, changes in dream patterns, nightmares, difficulty sleeping, nervousness, restlessness, anxiety, mental depression, rash, hives, itching, thinning or loss of scalp hair, difficulty urinating, and dryness and burning of the eyes. Clonidine increases the depressive effects of alcohol, barbiturates, sedatives, and tranquilizers. You should, therefore, avoid combining these different drugs.

There are many types of drug therapy provided for menopausal women. However, each woman has her own tolerance for medication. And, because you are taking these drugs for your own comfort, it is important to determine how their side effects will affect your life. It is only through self awareness that you will be able to feel assured that your treatment program is the best one for you.

Psychological approaches to the treatment of menopause:
Psychological approaches to treatment are those that focus on behaviour associated with menopause and techniques designed to modify this behaviour. There are three approaches used to deal

with menopausal symptoms or problems arising from menopause: general counseling about menopause; treatment of menopausal symptoms; and counseling for issues related to menopause.

General counseling about menopause

There are some women who like to be prepared for any new experience or who like to have an idea of the alternatives that can be available to them. General counseling, then, can provide women approaching or experiencing menopause with general information about menopause, what kinds of symptoms they may experience, and some alternative treatments that are available to help them. Counseling can also be effective in reducing symptoms of mild depression, irritability, anger, frustration, and/or in overcoming feelings that the menopause is a very distressing time. Therefore, imparting knowledge, giving advice about coping with minor problems, and being a supportive, listening ear are the prime purposes of a counselor.

General counseling is usually done by a general practitioner, gynecologist, other medical practitioner or a knowledgeable mental health worker. Very often it is carried out over one session or at the most a few.

Treating menopausal symptoms

Sometimes women try to alleviate their menopausal symptoms through psychological approaches rather than using drugs. They may, for example, be trying to deal with their hot flashes, headaches, backaches, general tension, and anxiety. But, in this case, it is not a symptom complex that requires treatment, but unique symptoms or one aspect of a symptom. For example, there are a series of behavioural techniques that have been shown to be useful in helping to reduce anxiety. Such approaches are:

- *Biofeedback* — With biofeedback the woman has electrodes attached to her skin that measure either heart rate, blood pressure or moisture or sweat on the skin. These measures provide the woman with immediate and direct feedback about her level of tension. Once the woman is trained to read the measurement, which will give her an idea of how stressed she is, she can then be taught how to lower the level of stress by concentrating on stress reduction or by using other relaxation methods such as slowing down her breathing. The important part of this technique is developing the woman's awareness of her level of tension and what it feels like to reduce it.

- *Relaxation techniques* — There are a variety of relaxation methods that can be hepful in reducing stress. With some methods the woman is trained to learn to use more relaxed deep breathing. Others involve the use of teaching the systematic contraction and relaxation of different parts of the body, such as tightening your hands as much as you can, then letting go and relaxing. This method also includes training in increased awareness of what tension and relaxation feel like.

- *Hypnosis* — Much of what people know about hypnosis seems to come from watching professional hypnotists make a willing participant from the audience act like a chicken or a dog. Actually, hypnosis is a very useful technique. It is not a method used to take away control from the person. It is, however, very useful in training women to be more relaxed. Some people think of hypnosis as being concentrated attention. Others compare it to an altered state of consciousness. In this state of heightened concentration, it is easier to train a woman to be more relaxed. People differ in their ability to go into deeper states of hypnosis. They also differ in their comfort with this technique. With hypnosis, it is possible to use suggestions or imagery to assist in the relaxation or to help remove some symptoms. Training in self-hypnosis allows the woman to use the technique whenever she feels she needs it.

- *Imagery* — Training in the use of imagery can take place either with or without hypnosis. It involves having the woman close her eyes and imagine a scene. It can be used for relaxation by having the woman imagine a scene that is associated in her mind with relaxation. When she becomes tense, she can use this image to facilitate relaxation. This technique can also be used to imagine a scene that will produce an effect that is the opposite to the one you want to get rid of. For example, some researchers have used imagery with women with hot flashes. They have trained the women to imagine they are in a cold, snowy setting. The women then use the images of coldness to reduce some of the effects of hot flashes.

- *Behavioural rehearsal* — This method can be used to help a woman cope with a difficult situation by having her rehearse in her mind the bothersome situation and by helping her at each step to find a solution so she can better handle the total situation and reduce the stress associated with it.

- *Assertiveness training* — This technique is also used to rehearse a situation in which the woman feels unassertive. The woman acts out alternatives in which she is more assertive to help her deal with each aspect of the situation. This method can be used to reduce anxiety that results from a lack of assertiveness in family or work situations or dealing with her physician in a satisfying and expressive way.

- *Induced anger* — This method involves training a woman who has problems in expressing or handling her anger to produce the image of an anger-arousing situation. She is then taught how to express her anger with appropriate behaviour and language. As she learns to express her anger appropriately, the anxiety associated with the anger is usually reduced.

These behavioural techniques are used usually by psychologists or hypnotherapists. They tend to be relatively short-term forms of therapy.

Counseling for issues or symptoms related to menopause

Some of the issues or symptoms associated with menopause can be more problematic for women. For these women a longer, more in-depth form of counseling or psychotherapy is helpful. Drs. Mary and Michael Dosey found that the women who sought counseling tended to perceive the menopausal process as unpleasant, both emotionally and physically.

Counseling can be an appropriate form of treatment for women when their menopausal symptoms are sufficiently intense to the degree that it interferes with their life, when menopause is associated with other stressful life events, or when a woman has had long-standing problems that she has not dealt with before but becomes more aware of during menopause.

Symptoms which interfere with life

For a small percentage of women, some of the symptoms that seem to be associated with menopause, such as depression, can become of sufficient intensity that they interfere with their lives. For a few other women, issues such as loss of femininity, problems with self esteem and loss of identity, become more crucial at this time. Women with these kinds of problems seem to benefit from more long-term counseling and support.

Stressful life events and menopause

In a number of recent studies, Drs. Cooke and Greene studied the relationship between life events and symptoms at the climacterium. They examined both what they called miscellaneous, or non-specific, and exit stress. Exit stress is caused by the children leaving home or parents dying. They found the relationship between life events and symptoms to be a very complex one, depending on the nature of the life events and the type of symptoms. Cooke and Greene discovered that women can become more vulnerable to miscellaneous, or non-specific, stress during this time, even if they had been able to deal with these stressors at an earlier age. Psychological symptoms during the climacterium were directly related to the degree of miscellaneous stress being experienced. Somatic symptoms during the menopause were affected by a combination of both kinds of life events. Menopause does not occur in a vacuum but is affected by the other events in a woman's life. For some women the degree to which the menopausal symptoms are bothersome will depend on what else is happening in their lives.

The relationship of menopausal symptoms to other symptomotologies

A small number of women have a more difficult time during menopause because their symptoms are very intense. We do not know enough to be able to determine whether these women differ in terms of their hormonal changes or whether their problems are more psychologically based. My feeling is that for some women, both may be true. Probably the major symptom that would bring a woman to a therapist during menopause is depression.

For other women, menopause seems to stir up or encourage feelings of loss or problems with self esteem, that may or may not have been present prior to this event. For example, some women associate reproduction with femininity. At menopause, the loss of femininity can then become an issue. For others, a history of problems that may include low self esteem, marital difficulties, conflict within the family, anxiety, fears, or loss of interest in sex may become more critical or more obvious at the time of menopause. For example, a woman who has used the excuse of fear of pregnancy or the requirements of child rearing to avoid sex has to deal with that issue at menopause.

Psychotherapy or counseling, then, is used for many purposes: support; developing coping strategies; teaching ways of developing social support networks; encouraging self awareness and expression; clarifying values; helping to focus on new goals; making the woman more aware of her strengths rather than focusing on her weaknesses; helping to minimize and eliminate feelings of anxiety, inadequacy, and depression; helping to generate alternatives; working through problems associated with the perception of menopause as a time of loss; helping menopausal widowed or divorced women to deal with loneliness, grief, and separation; assisting women to deal with their own sexuality and marital or family problems.

There are many different types of psychotherapy. They differ in the theoretical framework that is the basis of the approach. For example, psychoanalytic therapists follow the work of Sigmund Freud and focus on early childhood experiences as the basis of later problems. Cognitive restructuring approaches focus on restructuring the way in which people see their problems and ways of coping with them. Behaviour modification techniques help people learn new ways of dealing with situations. These are only a few. You may also have heard of Gestalt therapy and non-directive techniques. Some therapists use combinations of different types of approaches, depending on the type of problems with which they are working.

In addition, therapies can differ depending on whether they work with an individual, group, family, or couple. The therapies also stress different techniques, such as insight, free expression of feelings, role playing, assertiveness, communication skills, and others.

There are many different types of therapy available for the menopausal woman. Every woman differs in the kind of therapy that she needs and that she finds most satisfactory.

The use of psychotherapy is sometimes very useful in conjunction with drug therapy. Some problems are the result of both biological and psychological stress. This is the reason an individual assessment of your needs is so important. If you are seeking therapy, you would be wise to make sure you have been checked thoroughly to discover if there is any physical basis for your problems.

Psychotherapy is available through private clinicians and mental health workers in mental health centers, hospitals, and women's support clinics.

Who gives therapy?
Psychiatrists, psychologists, social workers, and physicians are some of the mental health workers who do psychotherapy. Check

the professional's title and qualifications before making a decision about a therapist.

How do I know if counseling is for me?
For the majority of women, menopause and its associated problems will not require therapy. However, if you are trying to decide whether therapy would be appropriate for you, some of these criteria might help.

- Do you feel that your anxiety level or depression is interfering with your life?
- Are you experiencing life events that you would like to talk about with someone who can give you a more objective opinion?
- Has counseling been suggested to you by a medical practitioner or someone whose opinion you trust?
- Do you feel you would like some support in making some major decisions?
- Have you had a long-standing problem that you have become more attuned to because of menopause?
- Are you concerned that your menopausal symptoms are due to psychological causes?
- Do you feel that you have been under considerable stress lately in addition to experiencing menopausal symptoms?
- Are you having problems dealing with aging that you would like to discuss?
- Do you find that you are consistently overreacting to even small problems?
- Do you feel you have been very hard on yourself lately and tend to focus primarily on the negative things in your life?

Selecting a therapist
- Consult someone you know and trust, such as your physician, who knows a number of therapists and would give you a reference.
- If you do not know someone who can give you a referral, then look in the yellow pages. You might want to call someone near you. Ask them to describe their therapeutic approach, how long they usually see clients for counseling, and the cost. Check whether their services are covered by your insurance.
- Many of the professional associations have a referral guide in which they list professionals and their areas of expertise. Check your local library.

- Make sure you are comfortable with your therapist. It is really important that you can discuss any topic with the person you see. If you are not comfortable after a few sessions, try someone else.
- Ensure that the type of approach the therapist uses makes sense to you.
- Check that the therapist seems knowledgeable about menopause.
- Select a therapist who seems to have a flexible approach. For example, is the therapist willing to do family counseling in addition to your own individual counseling?

The whole topic of selecting a therapist is a very complex one and I have only mentioned a few of the things you might want to think about when making your choice. There are consumers' guides to choosing therapists and you would be very wise to consult one of these.

Some hints about therapy
- The more informed you are about your symptoms, the more helpful you can be in the determination of the problem and the best type of therapy.
- If you are keeping a record of your menopausal symptoms, you will be able to separate the problems that seem related to menopause from those that are more influenced by other aspects of your life.
- If you are having problems with someone in your family, keeping notes about what is happening can help when you see the therapist.
- Be honest with yourself and with your therapist.
- If you write down some of your concerns before you go to the therapist, you will find it is easier to remember some of the details you wanted to cover or questions you wanted to ask.
- If you go for counseling and find you are embarrassed to discuss some issues, such as sexuality, it might help to admit you are embarrassed and discuss this first.

Natural treatments for menopause
In addition to the treatments described above, there are a series of natural treatments that are used for menopausal symptoms, such as the use of herbs, diet, vitamin supplements, and exercise. Before trying any of these more natural methods you would probably be wise to:

- Consult a physician and discuss your state of health, individual needs, and her/his opinion about the treatment program you would like to follow.
- In some cases you may want to get a second opinion from another physician or, perhaps, a dietician or pharmacologist or some other expert in nutrition and/or exercise. Not all physicians are knowledgeable about, or interested in, the use of nutrition, vitamins, and/or exercise as a form of treatment.
- Read as much as you can about the different treatments before starting on your own individual program. If you read simply from one source you may be misled. There is, for example, a case reported where someone followed a vitamin program recommended in one book and had a severe toxic reaction.
- Make sure your state of health is regularly monitored when following any program.

Herbal treatments
Ginseng and other types of herbs have been suggested as being potentially helpful for the menopausal woman. Some of the possible applications of ginseng to menopausal women have been described in a book by Barbara and Gideon Seaman. The Seamans based their information on a summary of research findings and on their own experiences in working with a number of menopausal women. They noted that ginseng is the "common name for several species of *Panax* herbs (its scientific name means panacea) belonging to the family *Aralicaeae*." It has been used in the Orient for thousands of years for the treatment of symptoms associated with aging. The Seamans commented that much of the research has used animals as subjects. However, they reported some of the Soviet research on humans demonstrated a relationship between the use of ginseng preparations and increased physical and mental efficiency, improved accuracy and concentration, and prevention of fatigue.

With regard to menopausal symptoms, ginseng has been used for hot flashes. "In our experience," the Seamans write, "women suffering from hot flashes take from ten days to six weeks to benefit from ginseng; two weeks is average before some effects are noticed. Some women with flashes do not benefit at all, but most say that (a) their flashes are gone or greatly diminished, or (b) they feel generally stronger and more resistant — they still get some flashes but do not feel 'knocked out' by them." They also indicate that other physicians have used ginseng, vitamin E, and dietary measures to treat hot flashes.

In addition to ginseng, Barbara and Gideon Seaman reported that two other herbs are used: goldenseal and Fo-ti-tieng. "Goldenseal is a traditional cure for night sweats of any origin, while Fo-ti-tieng is considered, by some herbalists, to be more of a specific for women than ginseng and the other products. . . . There seems little question that herbs of this general family prevent or relieve menopause symptoms in many women."

Ginseng comes in many forms: root, powder, teas, and capsules. The correct ginseng dosage varies with body weight. A woman weighing between 100 and 130 pounds should take one gram (1,000 mg). More is required if the woman is heavier. They also stated that "as a rule, ginseng is most effective when taken on an empty stomach, before or between meals, but not right after. It should not be taken simultaneously with vitamin C, which may weaken or neutralize its effects. Orientals also believe that the following foods should be avoided for three hours after taking ginseng: pineapple, tomato, grapefruit, lemon, orange, carrot, turnip. Vitamin E, however, and alcohol are believed to increase its effectiveness."

There are many ginseng products on the market and it is difficult to know the concentration of the herb in some of them. The Seamans suggest, therefore, that you buy ginseng from a health food store or pharmacy that you know and trust.

There are still many contradictory comments written about the use and effectiveness of ginseng. It is important to remember that herbal medications are also drugs and need to be used with considerable care. In Jane Brody's book, *The New York Times Guide to Personal Health*, she outlined several points that have been made about the use of herbal compounds, which include herbal teas:

- Often the side effects of these drugs are not reported.
- They are often sold in health food stores and are accompanied by books, pamphlets, magazines, and charts which contain information on health benefits, the validity of which is open to question.
- It is very difficult to know how herbal medications interact with other prescription drugs. "People with chronic ailments should tell their physician of any use of herbal preparations."
- Sometimes people requiring medical care will use herbal medications instead of the more appropriate drug treatment.
- Some people can be allergic to the teas made from different herbs.

- According to Dr. Der Manerosian, some medicinal teas such as mistletoe, shave grass, and sassafras, are too dangerous to be on the shelves.

In general, most of the popular herbal teas can be helpful and are used by people who cannot drink caffeine. The point is, however, that we should be very careful about anything that we ingest and make sure that we do not use large quantities. If there is a reaction, stop using the herb immediately.

Susan Flamholtz Trien in her book, *Change of Life: The Menopause Handbook*, also discussed the use of herbal teas for menopausal symptoms. She noted that herbs could be potent and some even toxic. She quoted a naturopath who suggested "two or three cups of herbal teas a day aren't likely to hurt you, but if you wish to experiment with various herbs you should do so under the supervision of an experienced physician or herbalist."

She listed the herbs that have been reported as being helpful in dealing with hot flashes including sarsaparilla, licorice, red raspberry, cramp bark, black cohosh, damiana, don quai, ginseng, squaw vine, and false unicorn root. These herbs are supposed to contain estrogen and stimulate the body to produce its own female hormones. She also suggested that a hot cup of herbal tea can be soothing before bedtime. "Herbs such as chamomile, scullcap, valerian root, hops, passion flower, and rosehips are especially good for calming the nerves, according to one health food store manager."

Nutrition and Menopause
For the menopausal woman, information about nutrition can help maintain good health, deal with the additional stress on the body during this time of change and in treating menopausal symptoms.

- Make sure you eat a balanced diet, which means eating from the four food groups; the meat group, the fruit and vegetable group, the milk group, and the grain group. You might want to refer to a couple of good nutrition books to find the amount of each group that is right for you.
- Read labels before buying and eating foods. Many of the foods have additives and preservatives that are not good for you.
- Become food conscious. Try keeping track of your own food intake so you can see for yourself, what your own eating habits are. From there you can plan changes that are best for you.

- Drink plenty of water. A woman I know carries a thermos of ice water. She has several drinks of ice water a day, which she finds both refreshing and healthy.
- Cut down on junk food. They are obviously low in nutrients. For many of us this may mean changing our life style. For example, it is so easy to pick up something on the way home when we are tired after work or to succumb to the demands of a teenager who wants pizza for dinner several nights a week.
- Check with your physician, a nutritionist, or dietitian before making any drastic changes in your diet. Each person has specific needs. Be wary of commercial diets; many do not suit your own individual nutritional needs.
- There are many exciting cookbooks on the market that present nutritional food in interesting ways.
- Lower your salt intake. Higher levels of salt intake have been related to hypertension, high blood pressure, and retention of water in the body tissues. For women, the retention of water has been associated with symptoms of premenstrual tension. To help reduce some of these symptoms, it would probably help to go on a low salt diet for at least the latter half of your menstrual cycle.
- Be aware of the fiber content in your diet. Fiber is the part of the food that is not digested by the body. Some examples of foods containing fiber are coarse bran, unpeeled fruits, oatmeal, sesame seeds, and whole grain breads. It is clear that fiber serves many useful purposes for the body. However, there is still considerable debate about exactly what it does. In spite of this, fiber is an important part of your diet and usually not enough is included in the average meals.
- Because a nutrient is good for you does not mean that high amounts of it will be even better. Read food guides and try not to overdo on any type of nutrient.
- Be aware of the cholesterol content of different foods. There are many food guides that will tell you the amount of cholesterol and calories indifferent kinds of food. You would also be wise to have your cholesterol level checked on a regular basis. This can be done by a blood test. If your level is above 200 milligrams per 100 milliliters of blood serum, you would benefit from cutting back on your intake of saturated fats and cholesterol. The American Heart Association recommends that the daily intake of cholesterol not exceed 300 milligrams. Most of us eat around 600 milligrams of cholesterol daily. The foods highest in cholesterol are eggs, red meat, seafood, and organ foods.

General Health

Good nutrition is important for the general health of menopausal women in several ways: it helps to maintain an optimal level of energy and ability to work efficiently; it increases the resistance to infection and disease; and it helps in the repairing of damage or injury to the body. There are many books and articles that have been written telling us about the proper amounts and kinds of nutrients we should consume. In Canada, our food requirements are listed in the Recommended Nutrient Intake for Canadians, and in the United States, the National Academy of Sciences developed the Recommended Dietary Allowances (RDA). The Canadian Recommended Nutrient Intakes guide describes the vitamin and mineral daily requirements for each sex and age group. One of the problems with using the guide is that it assumes that menopausal women have the same dietary requirements as other women. Many researchers suggest that this is not the case. For example, the guide suggests that women over 50 years of age should take 800 mg of calcium per day. However, many researchers agree that for the menopausal woman this amount is not enough. Drs. Cutler, Garcia and Edwards stated that since less dietary calcium is absorbed into the body from the digestive tract with aging, the amount of calcium you might need at menopause will depend on your unique metabolic requirements. They recommend taking about 1,000 mg per day to prevent bone loss.

Other researchers suggest that women should take 1,500 mg per day. Cutler, Garcia and Edwards also cautioned that you can take too much calcium, which may lead to calcification of the arterial areas (promoting arteriosclerosis) and kidney stones. According to their survey of the research, women consume less than half of the calcium they need. Many researchers feel that nutritional requirements change with age.

To improve the general health of menopausal women, here are some general suggestions:

- There seems to be an even greater need for good nutrition at menopause, since it is a time when the body is under more stress.
- When you are older, you tend to be less active and take longer to metabolize fats. Your ability to absorb vitamins and minerals from food is also less efficient. Therefore, you need fewer calories and more nutritious foods.

* The Recommended Nutrient Intakes for Canadians is currently under revision.

- Many women in the menopausal years become concerned about the increase in their weight. Some researchers suggest that with menopause many women gain about 10 to 15 pounds. In our society we seem so oriented to the slender woman. The chart by the Metropolitan Life Insurance Company will give you an idea of the ideal weight for women for their height. You may be surprised by the average weights that are reported. In the menopausal group, there are many advantages to being slightly heavier: you are likely to produce more estrogen; you are less likely to develop osteoporosis, partly because the heavier mass puts more of a stress on the bones, thus developing more bone mass. Also, some researchers find that heavier women have fewer problems with hot flashes.

- If you try to lose weight at menopause, it seems easier at this

TABLE 2

Metropolitan Heights and Weight Tables

MEN					WOMEN				
Height		Small Frame	Medium Frame	Large Frame	Height		Small Frame	Medium Frame	Large Frame
Feet	Inches				Feet	Inches			
5	2	128-134	131-141	138-150	4	10	102-111	109-121	118-131
5	3	130-136	133-143	140-153	4	11	103-113	111-123	120-134
5	4	132-138	135-145	142-156	5	0	104-115	113-126	122-137
5	5	134-140	137-148	144-160	5	1	106-118	115-129	125-140
5	6	136-142	139-151	146-164	5	2	108-121	118-132	128-143
5	7	138-145	142-154	149-168	5	3	111-124	121-135	131-147
5	8	140-148	145-157	152-172	5	4	114-127	124-138	134-151
5	9	142-151	148-160	155-176	5	5	117-130	127-141	137-155
5	10	144-154	151-163	158-180	5	6	120-133	130-144	140-159
5	11	146-157	154-166	161-184	5	7	123-136	133-147	143-163
6	0	149-160	157-170	164-188	5	8	126-139	136-150	146-167
6	1	152-164	160-174	168-192	5	9	129-142	139-153	149-170
6	2	155-168	164-178	172-197	5	10	132-145	142-156	152-173
6	3	158-172	167-182	176-202	5	11	135-148	145-159	155-176
6	4	162-176	171-187	181-207	6	0	138-151	148-162	158-179

Weights at ages 25-59 based on lowest mortality. Weight in pounds according to frame (in indoor clothing weighing 5 lbs., shoes with 1-inch heels).

Weights at ages 25-59 based on lowest mortality. Weight in pounds according to frame (in indoor clothing weighing 3 lbs., shoes with 1-inch heels).

time to lose calcium, even though you are taking calcium supplements.

- Since the chances of cardiovascular problems seems to increase over 50 years of age, it is probably a time when it is more important to very carefully watch your cholesterol intake. This means that you limit the number of eggs per week to three, the amount of lean red meat you eat, and the seafood and whole milk products that you consume.

- Try to limit the amount of refined sugars, white flour, alcohol, caffeine, chocolate, red meat, butter, cream, and salt that you consume.

- There is a general concern about the use of sugars after menopause because of their suggested relationship with increased cholesterol.

- Many diet conscious menopausal women, in an attempt to lower their weight, are limiting their calorie intake. The concern is that in lowering the calories, they are limiting important nutrients.

- According to Rosetta Reitz, a healthier diet results in a later, easier menopause.

- In *The New Our Bodies, Ourselves* , the authors indicate that menopausal women do not absorb as much protein as they did previously. This means that it is important for menopausal women to be concerned about their level of protein intake, but not those associated with increased animal fat. On the other hand, there is some suggestion that high protein diets can cause a loss of calcium from the body. This will give you an idea of the complexities involved in the whole area of nutrition for the menopausal woman.

- Fiber in vegetables, fruit, and whole grain will help constipation and reduce cholesterol.

- It would appear that the optimal diet for the menopausal woman would be high in vegetables, whole grain, fruits, and foods high in calcium.

- Try to avoid canned or pickled vegetables since they are high in salt content.

- The kind of meat you eat during the menopausal years should be lean and have minimal cholesterol content. Also, the amount of red meat you eat should be cut down. Try eating a four-ounce steak when you go to a restaurant. If you can eat chicken, with the skin removed, lean veal, and fish instead of other red meats, do so.

Specific types of foods can also be useful for specific menopausal symptoms.

Osteoporosis : Many researchers have noted that diets with increased amounts of calcium, vitamin D, and sodium fluoride seem to help prevent and lessen bone loss. But it is again important to remember that each of these can become toxic if taken in excessive amounts. Calcium seems to be the most critical nutrient related to bone loss. However, some of the foods that are high in calcium are also high in phosphorus which, some suggest, draws calcium away from the bones. Barbara and Gideon Seaman list some foods, such as turkey, ham, pork, fried potatoes, bread, processed cheese, nuts, crackers, and soft drinks, that fit into this category. Again, this shows the incredible complexity of trying to balance your nutritional needs, which is why the help of a doctor or nutritionist is so necessary. According to the Seamans, to prevent osteoporosis, your calcium intake must be balanced against the proper amounts of both magnesium (so the calcium stays in your bones and is not excreted) and phosphorus. Many scientists have suggested that the intake of calcium should be roughly about twice the amount of magnesium and at least equal to the amount of phosphorus. To prevent and control osteoporosis with your diet the amount of alcohol and caffeine should also be limited.

Hot flashes : Alcohol, caffeine, and spicy foods have all been suggested to be triggers for hot flashes for some women and, therefore, should be avoided as much as possible during this time. Foods containing vitamins E and C have been considered as helpful in the prevention and treatment of hot flashes, although for many women, vitamin treatment has not been shown to be effective in controlling the hot flashes.

Bloating : There are many foods that are considered to be natural diuretics and may help with the retention of water in the tissues. Some suggested foods are celery, parsley, watermelon, grapes, fresh pineapple, canteloupe, asparagus, and cucumbers. However, the problem with any diuretic, either natural or synthetic, is that they have been associated with the reduction of potassium and zinc in the body. Again, a balanced diet is necessary.

Constipation : Fiber is a natural laxative. However, too much fiber in our diets can cause gas and intestinal discomfort.

Sleeping problems : Tryptophane, found in warm milk and some meats, is thought to have sedative effects. Try warm milk before going to bed if you are having some sleeping problems. (It also helps to focus your mind on positive things before trying to sleep. If you start to worry, try to focus on something pleasant).

Irritability: The B vitamins have been related to reducing stress and depression. Some physicians believe that irritability and depression can be a result of the balance between sodium and potassium. Eating foods that contain these nutrients is certainly better than taking tranquilizers.

Osteoarthritis: While the Arthritis Foundation does not feel that arthritis can be helped by nutrition, there are some researchers who are more open to the possible effects of such nutrients as niacin, pantothenic acid, riboflavin, vitamin A, vitamin B6, magnesium, calcium, phosphate, and other minerals.

Healthy skin: Several vitamins have been related to healthy skin. These include vitamin A, B12 and biotin, B2, D, and pantothenic acid. Some researchers feel that if you are having problems with your skin, you should check your diet to ensure you are not deficient in these vitamins.

As you can imagine, much research is needed before we can accept any of these nutritional treatments. However, it is clear that with menopause, women need to become very aware of what and how much they are eating and much more conscious of the nutrients in food. It makes considerable sense that if we can find natural ways of preventing or treating menopausal symptoms, it would be much better than the use of medication. Hopefully in the near future we will know more about nutrition as a treatment for menopause.

Vitamin and mineral supplements
In addition to the vitamins and minerals found in food sources, supplements are also available. These come in various forms: tablets, capsules, liquid, powder, drops, or ointment. They are sold in drug and health food stores.

Vitamin supplements can either be natural or synthetic. A natural vitamin has as its source either a plant or animal. Synthetic vitamins, on the other hand, have the same chemical structure as the natural vitamins, but are produced artificially by the synthesis of simpler materials. However, there may be other factors such as minerals, proteins, or other vitamins that are in the natural nutrient but not the synthetic compound. Also, artificial coloring or flavouring may be in the synthetic form.

The Nutrition Almanac describes another form of nutrient supplement: co-natural vitamins. These contain a combination of natural and synthetic vitamins. The synthetic nutrients are added to increase the potency or stability of the natural vitamin and to standardize the amount of nutrients per capsule. One way to detect a synthetic nutrient is from the label, since they often contain a salt form that is used to increase the stability of the nutrient. The salt forms used are listed as palmatate, sulfate, nitrate, hydrocholoride, chloride, succinate, bitartrate, acetate, and gluconate.

In making decisions about nutrient supplements you might want to consider the following:

- Nutrient supplements became popular when people started to be concerned about the soil in which the fruits and vegetables were grown, in addition to the types of fertilizers used. However, most researchers agree that vitamins and minerals from foods are the best source of vitamins. If you eat a well-balanced meal, it is unlikely you will need vitamin supplements.

- Vitamin supplements are useful when you have been under extra stress or illness, have a deficiency condition, do not eat properly, or are not absorbing efficiently the vitamins and minerals from your foods. Some feel that in winter, when fresh fruits and vegetables are not as readily available and when the weather conditions produce potential stress on the body, that it is good to take a multivitamin. Others believe very strongly in the preventative aspects of taking vitamin C to avoid colds.

- Vitamins and minerals interact with each other. To maximize the absorption of a nutrient, you often need to take it in combination with others.

- Keep in mind that vitamins and minerals are drugs and have side effects and levels of toxicity. Become familiar with the possible side effects before using them.

- Some vitamins have been suggested to be counterindicated if you have certain health problems. For example, it is suggested by some writers to avoid vitamin E in large doses if you have high blood pressure. You would be wise to check with a medical practitioner before starting to take different nutrients.

- Make sure you read the labels and look for such things as artificial coloring or flavoring.
- If you are taking any other kinds of medication, you would probably be wise to consult with your physician before starting supplements.
- Even if you are taking vitamin supplements, your diet should still be the primary source of nutrients.
- Some vitamins are toxic in large doses. For example, large amounts of vitamins A and D are toxic. Excessive zinc can aggravate an otherwise inconsequential copper deficiency. Too much phosphorous may interfere with the body's use of calcium. Excess vitamin B6 can induce depressive symptoms. High doses of niacin can cause heart rhythm irregularities and gastrointestinal problems. Too much vitamin C has been related to kidney stones.
- It has been suggested that with the exception of vitamin E it does not make much difference whether you use the natural or synthetic form of a vitamin or mineral.
- Most vitamins should be taken with meals. Fat soluble vitamins seem to be best absorbed when taken with fatty foods.

Nutritional supplements and menopause
While much more research is necessary, some writers recommend taking nutrient supplements for menopausal symptoms:

- The use of a multivitamin is recommended by some as a way to help with a general feeling of well-being.
- For hot flashes, both vitamin C and E have been suggested, although the research indicates that for many women the vitamins are not particularly helpful.
- For heavy bleeding, vitamin A and iron tablets have been given.
- To help with the general stress to the body caused by menopause, some women have used the vitamin B6 and magnesium. Some believe that magnesium can help muscles and nerves relax and is safer than tranquilizers.
- Some women have taken vitamin E to increase their libido or sex drive. The research, again, does not support this treatment as being effective.

- It is recommended to some women who have been taking hormone replacement therapy for a year or more to take vitamins B6 and E.

- For menopausal symptoms, the most information is available on the use of calcium supplements to help prevent osteoporosis or stop further bone loss if a woman already has the disease. Because at menopause the calcium requirements increase to 1,000 to 1,500 mg, calcium supplements are often necessary. It is important, however, to make sure that you balance your daily intake between your diet and supplements. Excessive levels of calcium have been related to calcification in the arteries, which can lead to arteriosclerosis. There are different types of calcium supplements that differ in the percentage of calcium they contain. According to Wendy Smith and Dr. Cohn, calcium carbonate tablets are 40 percent calcium, calcium lactate 13 percent, calcium gluconate only 9 percent. They also noted that several brands of antacid, the ones without aluminum, have as much calcium as calcium carbonate. The possible side effects of calcium carbonate tablets at high dosages are constipation and flatulence. Ms. Smith and Cr. Cohn suggest that if problems occur, calcium gluconate is less constipating. They also reported a 1982 study that found lead contamination in bone meal and dolomite. It is, therefore, wise to avoid these. As we age, we also need more vitamin D to help with the proper absorption of calcium. Many researchers have recommended 15 minutes a day of exposure to sunlight. It may, however, be necessary at this time to increase your dietary amount of vitamin D or to take supplements. Since vitamin D can become toxic rather quickly, it is best to stick to the 400 IUs per day. Some writers discuss the value in taking magnesium with the calcium in a ratio of two amounts of calcium to one of magnesium. Some also feel that phosphorus intake should equal but not exceed the amount of calcium consumed.

Vitamin and mineral supplements can certainly be helpful to the menopausal woman. It is clear, though, that they should be used with considerable care. You would be wise to seek professional advice before starting on a treatment program to make sure that it meets your needs.

Exercise
We all know that exercise is important for us at every stage of our lives, but many women would like to know how it can help them

during menopause. For the menopausal woman, there are two kinds of benefits from exercise: those relating to a state of general health and those more specifically appropriate to menopausal symptoms.

General health
At any age, exercise has been associated with a general feeling of well being. Women who are in better condition seem to have more energy and feel better about themselves. It also can help stress reduction because any kind of exercise seems to use some of the nervous energy. Exercise also benefits your sleeping and bowel functioning, as well as lowering your heart rate; controlling cholesterol and blood pressure levels; and improving your appearance, in terms of tighter muscles, a look of increased vitality, and better utilization of calories. Barbara and Gideon Seaman also felt that exercise was essential for aging bones, the cardiovascular system and helps with a program of therapeutic nutrition. They also stated that there was convincing evidence that ligaments can be strengthened by almost any reasonable sort of exercise. They described two new studies that demonstrated that even moderate exercise of 30 minutes, three times a week, can provide protection against coronary attacks.

The New Our Bodies, Ourselves attributes lower blood pressure and reduced atherosclerosis, risks of heart attack and stroke, arthritis, emphysema, and osteoporosis to a sensible exercise program. The authors stated that there seems to be evidence that with exercise the blood rushes to the skin, bringing with it extra nutrients and causing the skin's temperature to rise. They felt the collagen content then increases and the skin actually thickens and becomes more elastic and less wrinkled.

Menopausal symptoms
In *The New Our Bodies, Ourselves*, the authors suggest moderate exercise is necessary for good health. "In fact, exercise, especially aerobic exercise, can produce in midlife many (if not all) of the things that the estrogen literature of the early seventies claimed would follow estrogen intake, including (for some women) reduction of hot flashes." While the relationship between exercise and hot flashes is a topic requiring more research, exercise can both help to prevent and treat osteoporosis. Exercises that involve weight-bearing have been related to increased bone density. In fact, many researchers feel that exercise is an important part of

both prevention and treatment of osteoporosis. According to Drs. Cutler, Garcia and Edwards, exercise in a certain area of the body will increase the bone mass in that area, although they described two studies that found that the bone mass in active compared to less active menopausal women failed to find the expected differences. While extremes of activity did relate to production of bone mass, varying amounts of activity within a normal range did not necessarily change the bone mass. However, regular exercise did promote greater muscle tone and mass. Again, more information is needed before we can have a clear understanding of the relationship between exercise and bone mass. For example, it is not clear how much exercise is required to increase bone mass. What does seem consistent is that there are a series of exercises that are more likely to be related to increased bone mass. Wendy Smith and Dr. Cohn included in their list of weight-bearing exercises: aerobic dancing, bicycling, calisthenics, canoeing, free-weight training, gymnastics, hiking, jogging, jumping rope, rowing, weight training on machines, and walking.

It is also clear that the exercises that are appropriate for the prevention and treatment of osteoporosis are very different. The types of exercise just described will help to promote bone mass and are, therefore, beneficial for the prevention of osteoporosis. If a woman has osteoporosis, she has to be very careful and selective in the types of exercise she does. Exercise is, however, still necessary and it is very important to select the right ones. There are specially designed programs for women with osteoporosis offered through some hospitals and women's clinics. The best type of exercise involves very easy stretching movements that are not strenuous. They are a very critical part of a program for any woman who has osteoporosis.

When you are planning an exercise program, there are several things you might keep in mind:

- Your general state of health and whether you have any type of health problem that might determine the type of exercise program you can do. For example, women with cardiovascular problems generally will not be able to participate in strenuous exercises.
- Your individual skills. Play to your strengths but don't ignore your weaknesses.
- Your prior history of exercise. Women who have been accustomed to regular strenuous exercises, such as tennis, will be

able to continue to use these exercises as part of their program when they are menopausal. If you have not been involved in regular exercising prior to menopause, it will be necessary to start any program very slowly.

• If you are planning an exercise program in your menopausal years, you would be wise to consult an expert in the field who can take into consideration your health, skills, and previous exercising history to plan a program that would best meet your needs.

• Check with your physician before starting any exercise program and have a complete physical examination. You might want to ask her/him: are there are any exercises that would be beneficial for you, any exercises you should not do, how you will know if an exercise or exercise program is too difficult or potentially harmful for you and if the program you plan should include moving from one level of difficulty to another.

• The timing of a program should be set according to your own needs. Some women are better able to follow an exercise program if it is in a particular time of the day. It is better to set a consistent, regular time for any exercising so you will maximize the probability that you will continue it. You know your own life style and time demands, and an exercise program will only be followed if it fits both of these.

• Make some decisions about what type of program would best meet your individual needs. For example, you might want to ask yourself if you are more likely to enjoy and continue exercising if you: exercise by yourself or with others; enjoy competitive or noncompetitive sports; exercise out-of-doors or inside; do a particular kind of exercise; are in a structured program, exercise with or without music.

• Many types of exercise are available. Remember, start slowly. Find a good time in the day to exercise. Whatever you do should be at your level. Be wary of exercises on television that may be too strenuous, such as aerobic exercises. Try to make it fun; perhaps some of your friends can join you. Dress comfortably and make sure you have the proper equipment. It is important to improve your muscle tone and cardiovascular state and different exercises are designed for each of these; try not just to exercise only one part of your body. The way in which you breathe during exercising is also an essential part of any exercise programme. If due to health reasons you cannot participate in regular exercise programs, try walking.

- Never overexercise. Listen to your body. It will tell you when you have done too much.
- If you are bedridden for a long time, ask your doctor what kind of exercises you can do in bed. Immobilization is related to a loss of calcium from the bones.
- Exercise and relaxation can very easily get lost in a busy schedule. Make sure you allow time for them. They are important.

Information on exercising and special programs designed for women with specific health problems are available through books and different exercising clinics. No matter what you do, make sure you exercise regularly and your program is designed to your specific needs. The importance of exercising for menopausal women can not be overemphasized, even if it just consists of simple stretching movements.

Chapter Six

Coping with Menopause

Answers to the question *How do women cope with menopause?* indicated that a positive attitude, obtaining information from physicians or other sources, and being able to rely on the support of others are needed. Some specific recommendations are listed below.

- *Positive attitude*
  - "Take one day at a time."
  - "Accept it and cope with the process."
  - "Try to get through it with patience."
  - "Take it slow and let nature run its course."
  - "Most women who have a healthy attitude to life will go through menopause as just another phase in their cycle of life."
  - "You realize it won't last too long so you accept it as best you can. Some react much better than others."
  - "If the mother got through it with a positive attitude, so will the daughter."
  - "Keep active and interested in life and living. Do some sort of sport or exercise program."
  - "Accept it as a normal and healthy part of life."

- *Medical advice*
  - "Consult a medical practitioner to try and obtain the necessary health care."
  - "Get a good doctor's advice."
  - "If there are any problems they should consult a physician."
  - "Seek advice about estrogen and whether it is right for you."

- *Support*
  - "Get involved in a group with other women of the same age."
  - "Get the support and understanding of other women."
  - "Rely on your family and friends. A lot depends on how they treat you."

- *Get information*
  - "Read about what to expect."
  - "Some women have problems because they are ill-informed."

To summarize how women cope, one woman wrote, "Some flourish and some falter."

We still do not know enough to be able to predict with a high degree of accuracy which women may find menopause more or less easy or difficult. But we do know some of the symptoms that make a woman higher risk. It should be remembered, though, that because you are high risk does not mean you will necessarily get all the symptoms. Also, different women deal with the what seems to be a similar symptom in very different ways. Perhaps the way you can cope with symptoms will determine how they will affect you. Here some suggestions for coping with menopause:

Jim and Sally Comway discussed what they described as "actions for blooming." These include dreaming ("allow your mind to flow in different directions");: set goals; try new adventures; go back to school; give attention to your body; eat correctly; exercise; and relate. One could add to these comments to enjoy the "now" rather than being concerned about the future; realize that expectations set when you were young may be unrealistic goals; focus more on positive achievements and goals than on negative aspects. Added to these suggestions are the following:

- Menopause is a concrete sign of a time of change or re-evaluation. Use it as such and as a time to sort out your alternatives.
- The women I interviewed expected a great deal of themselves. They felt they should be able to cope with a family, work, social life, household duties, and anything else that arose in their lives. Not being able to handle all these things was associated with guilt and, sometimes, feelings of inadequacy. During menopause, women are also experiencing physical changes

that may or may not be disruptive and associated with aging. Perhaps by evaluating the kinds of pressures you are undergoing, you will be able to judge yourself using more appropriate criteria. Be fair to yourself and in doing so, you will probably realize that your reactions to most situations are very appropriate and should not be associated with feelings of guilt or inadequacy.

- Look for positive role models, women who are menopausal and enjoying it. It helps!

- Midlife can be a time that is the "Me" age for women when we can focus more on our own needs and goals. Many women stated that as they became middle-aged, they finally had more time for themselves. This may be the time to identify what your needs and goals are and plan to meet them.

- Bring menopause out of the closet. The more prepared you are for menopause, the easier the experience will probably be. If you have only limited information about menopause, you will be more likely to be open to the myths surrounding this topic. From both discussions with women and in their answers to the questionnaires, many commented that they were not interested or did not know about menopause because they were not there yet. These comments seem to reflect the attitude of society that menopause is a topic that should not be discussed until or unless the symptoms associated with it require attention. In fact, being prepared for this life event can be helpful for women. Some suggestions for ways of being prepared would be: to talk to other women about their feelings and experiences; to discuss with your physician what you, as an individual, might expect and what you can do to best help yourself; to read as much as you can about menopause from many different sources (for example, while you may not agree with the feminist philosophy, reading a book written by a feminist may be extremely helpful to you, or even though you disagree with a medical approach, reading something written by a physician may give you much useful knowledge); to join a support group where women discuss issues that pertain to themselves.

- Become more aware of your own attitudes that relate to issues relevant to the menopausal woman, such as how you feel about not being able to have any more children or whether you associate being menopausal with feelings of being less feminine. If you are aware of your attitudes then you can do something about them. With regard to your feelings about having more children, you may want to think about why. Is it, for example, that you like having young children around, or do you associate not being able to have children with aging or loss of femininity? Or are you in a new relationship and would like to be able to share that experience with your husband? If you can determine which of these is the main focus of your feelings then you can develop alternative ways of dealing with that concern. For example, if you like to spend time with young children you can spend more time with your grandchildren or volunteer to help out in a nursery program or assist a child who needs extra help at school. If your concern is about aging, try to focus on the positive aspects of it. If femininity is an issue, try to redefine what being feminine is and find activities that help to make you feel more feminine. If you want to be close to your husband, set aside time when you can enjoy being with each other. While these are just some suggestions, they are really intended to say that if you are more aware of yourself and your attitudes, then you can find alternative ways of satisfying your needs.

- As many writers have suggested, middle age can be a time of self awareness and self growth. Enjoy it!

Coping with the symptoms

- We know that many of the symptoms that are associated with menopause can also be present in other age groups. Therefore, if you know the history of your own symptoms, you will be better able to identify those that seem to be a result of, or have been intensified by, menopause. This should help both in your understanding your symptoms and in determining the best treatment.

- Remembering that menopausal symptoms are only transitory might make someone who is trying to cope with some unpleasant symptoms feel a little better. It might also be beneficial to think about the postmenopausal zest that has been described by women such as Margeret Mead.

- Try to identify your feelings about your menopausal symptoms. For example, understanding that you are concerned that your hot flashes are visible to others can lead to a way of dealing with that concern. Some women feel that hot flashes are visible when they are really not noticeable to others. Even if they are visible, some people may just admire your healthy complexion.

It might help to get some feedback from others. Or if you think it would make you feel better, make a joke about your flush when the visibility of it is particularly bothersome. Some women have suggested to try and think of the flush as being an enjoyable glow of excitement.

• Being aware of your reactions to situations, that is how you deal with unpredictability, how role models affect you, how you cope with new situations, might help you understand how you feel about menopause.

• Some women feel that having symptoms at menopause is neurotic. For example, some women are surprised when they become depressed for a short period of time during menopause and wonder if they are just overreacting or being neurotic. We just still do not know enough about the causes of menopausal symptoms so it is much better not to judge ourselves so harshly. Again, some information from your physician may help.

• If you recall, I described the comments of the woman who felt her symptoms were menopausal only to discover that she had a thyroid problem. This really does suggest that we should be careful not to jump to conclusions about symptoms that occur when we are in the menopausal age group.

• Avoid labeling yourself, or accepting the labels of others, as to what menopause is and means. The mother who has an adolescent son or daughter who is going through a difficult stage may be irritable, not because of menopause, but because of her family situation. Women's reactions to their symptoms may depend on how these symptoms are labeled by themselves, their family, physicians, and others.

• You will probably find it easier to cope with menopause if you think about what the positive changes are that can be associated with this time. Why not ask yourself what you see as being the positive changes and try to focus more on them?

• If you do have menopausal symptoms that are bothersome, decide what would be the best way to pamper yourself. By accepting yourself as a menopausal woman, with whatever changes come with that, the whole experience should be more positive.

• Some of the women with whom I spoke expressed considerable concern over their symptoms. There could be many reasons for their concern: the symptoms may be unpleasant; they could feel they will never stop; or they could be associated with concepts, such as aging, that the woman may not accept. Probably the best way to deal with these concerns is to, on the one hand, accept them and get enough information so you have an idea of why you have these symptoms and how long they might last.

- Allow yourself the flexibility of being irritable, angry, or whatever. Many women described to me feeling more irritable, but just ignoring it and getting on with their lives. If they overreacted to a situation, they did not let it bother them. If they felt angry, they did not assume it was necessarily menopausal but they made sure they expressed their anger in a way that was appropriate for them.

- Watch your general health. Being overtired or stressed because of other health problems will probably make it more difficult to tolerate menopausal symptoms.

- Try to avoid making major decisions at times when you are feeling down.

Social relationships

- Many women have recommended that maintaining satisfying relationships is important in adjusting to menopause. One woman described a group of four women, all of whom were in a similar age range and who were menopausal, who when they were fed up with themselves or their lives would call one of the other women to go for a long walk. She said they always felt better after both the exercise and being able to talk to someone.

- Make sure you do not cut yourself off from social contacts if you are not feeling up to par because of menopausal symptoms. Talking out your feelings usually helps and many of us have a tendency to avoid social contacts when we feel we cannot make a positive contribution. During menopause it will probably help to know you are not alone.

Work:

- As part of the whole process of re-evaluation that can go on during menopause and middle age, one of the things that you can reconsider is your work. If you are not working, you may want to think about what you would like to do. If you are working, you may decide that you would like to change positions, improve your skills, or go back to school. The important part of the process is realizing that this period in your life can be a time of tremendous growth.

Physical appearance
- Some women become very concerned about their appearance during middle age and menopause can make these concerns more apparent. For example, there are some women who do not like their graying hair, wrinkes, or changing body proportions. Others just accept these changes as natural and are not concerned about them. One woman commented to me that she had been quite upset about her wrinkles until she saw a television program in which a number of middle-aged women were on a panel discussing some topic. She was very impressed with the maturity, intelligence, knowledge, and personalities of these women and with the kind of role models they represented. After seeing the program she started to realize the growth potential of middle-aged women. With this realization, the wrinkles were no longer a negative sign but represented increasing maturity. How you perceive your own physical changes in middle age will depend on what you associate with these changes. If you do feel negative about them you can either try to refocus the way you think about them or you can decide how you want to change them, e.g., by coloring your hair, using makeup to conceal wrinkles, or cosmetic surgery. Just realizing there are many options open to you may make you feel better.

Management of symptoms
- One of the important aspects for menopausal women is to select medical practitioners who are familiar with menopausal symptoms. For example, with declining amounts of estrogen there can be changes in the mucosa (or tissues) lining not only the vagina but also the nose, eyes, and mouth. Therefore, if you are peri- or postmenopausal you would want to select a dentist who was familiar with the symptoms that could affect any dental work, such as dry mouth or thinning of the bone. A dentist who is aware of some of these problems can help you to monitor your condition, e.g., through bone loss. And, even if you do not have any problems, you will probably benefit from their understanding. You should also be able to ask how menopause affects a particular part of your body and how you can be best prepared. For example, you may want to ask your dentist if there is anything you should do to keep your teeth and gums in the best condition during the menopausal and post-menopausal period. The same principle would apply to the selection of an allergist, nutritionist, or psychotherapist.

- In selecting a physician, if you are menopausal, you may want to discuss with the physician her/his attitudes to estrogen replacement therapy, the use of vitamins, and diet. If you are the kind of person who wants to take an active role in deciding about your treatment you will need to know that your physician finds that acceptable. Also, you will probably want someone who is accessible and who will take the time to talk to you.
- During menopause it is important to keep active, both physically and mentally. Do the things that give you a feeling of accomplishment.

There are a number of questions you can ask yourself that may tie together the points I have just described:

What do I want to do?
    – What am I doing now? Am I satisfied with my life?
    – Do I want to do something else in my work, exercise, diet or study, with my family or friends?
    – Is there something I have wanted to do for a long time but have put off because I did not have the time?
    – Am I not trying something I want to do, like going back to school, because I am concerned I might not be able to do it well?
    – What alternatives are open to me?

How do I feel?
    – How do I feel about myself? Am I being fair in my evaluation?
    – Am I concerned about my changing appearance? If so, how can I best deal with my concern?
    – Would I like to change some of my characteristics? If so, how can I do this?
    – Do I share my feelings with others? If not, would it help me if I did?
    – With whom can I share my feelings?
    – Does my husband and/or children know how I feel? If not, what is the best way to tell them?
    – If I feel guilty about what my children are doing, is it justified?
    – How am I feeling about getting older?
    – How do I feel about becoming menopausal or my menopausal symptoms?

How can I handle my menopausal years with the least amount of stress?
- Do I understand what happens during menopause? If not, how can I get the information in the best way for me?
- Do I take time for myself?
- Am I expecting too much of myself or others?
- Am I expecting too little of myself or others? Am I underestimating myself?
- Do I have a support system?
- Do I need professional help in dealing either with my own or with my family's problems?

In answering these types of questions, it is possible to become more aware of yourself, your method of solving problems, and the kinds of things you might want to do to make your menopausal years less stressful and more satisfying.

What to ask your physician

Since every woman's experience of menopause is unique, it is very important that you play an active role in making decisions about the kind of treatment you will receive and that you very carefully choose the best physician who will meet your needs. Both in making decisions about the selection of your physician and in discussing the best type of treatment for you, you may want to consider the following:

• What is your physician's attitude to menopause? Does your physician follow more a medical model where menopause is considered an estrogen deficiency disease or is your physician more concerned about the psychological components?
• Does your physician follow a certain approach to treatment of menopausal symptoms? If so, is it one with which you agree?
• Does your physician take menopausal symptoms seriously, or is she/he apt to say "It's only menopausal"? Alternatively, does your physician see many of the symptoms of a middle-aged woman as being menopausal, when perhaps they are not?
• Is your physician interested in talking to you about menopause before you have any symptoms? Does your doctor tell you to wait and see what symptoms you have?
• When your physician prescribes a medication for you, does she/he also explain to you what the drug is, why you are taking it, and what the possible side effects are?

- Are you comfortable asking your physician about your symptoms and what they mean?
- Are you and your physician both comfortable discussing topics such as sexuality?
- Is your physician supportive?
- Will your physician discuss such issues as diet or taking vitamins?
- Does your physician refer you to a specialist when necessary?
- Does your physician explain your symptoms to you in sufficient detail that you understand what is involved?

I asked some women *what information they would want to know from their physician about menopause.* Here are some of their questions:

- "Is there anything in my medical history that would make me high risk for any kind of menopausal symptom?"
- "If I am at risk for any condition, such as osteoporosis, should I be watching my diet or taking any vitamin supplements?"
- "Is there any way I can prepare for menopause with my diet, an exercise program or vitamins?"
- "Will menopause affect how I look?"
- "Will I start to age faster after menopause?"
- "Will menopause affect my sex life?"
- "Will I start to grow hair on my face?"
- "Will I lose my brain power faster after menopause?"
- "What can I do to keep my skin from drying out?"
- "Will menopause affect my life so I will not have as much fun or will I feel stronger when I'm not having periods?"
- "Will estrogen help me?"
- "If I take estrogen am I more prone to cancer?"
- "What can I do or take so I do not have to take estrogen?"
- "What can I do if I have hot flashes and I cannot take estrogen? Are there other treatments available?"
- "How will I know if I need counseling to help me through menopause?"
- "When should I seek medical treatment?"
- "Will I gain or lose weight during menopause?"
- "Is it possible for me to become pregnant during menopause?"
- "Can I adjust the time when I will become menopausal, that is prolong or speed up?"

It is clear that women have many questions that they would like to discuss with their physicians. It is also evident that some physicians are more approachable than others. If you have questions to ask your physician, make sure you set aside enough time so you do not feel rushed and you have a chance to ask all your questions. It might help to write down your questions before you go to see your physician. Also, do not assume that your physician will remember your relevant history. They have many patients. You might want to remind him/her if you have had any problems in the past that might affect the type of symptoms or treatment that would be appropriate for you. If you are not satisfied with your physician's attitude, knowledge, or opinion with regard to your symptoms or treatment, see another doctor. Remember, it's your body.

Stress and menopause
How stressful menopause is for a woman will depend on many things:

- the symptoms she has and their type, number, frequency, duration, and intensity;
- her threshold for symptoms. Some women have a higher threshold for coping with symptoms than others. The lower the threshold the more stress will probably be associated with the symptoms;
- the support she has;
- the other sources of stress in her family, work, or social life;
- her ability to find appropriate advice or medical assistance;
- how she feels about menopause;
- whether her symptoms are affecting her ability to sleep;
- whether she feels comfortable sharing her feelings with others.

There are several potential sources of stress during menopause. Some researchers suggest that stress may affect menopausal symptoms such as hot flashes. Only future research will tell us if this is true.

If you feel stressed during menopause, it is not unusual. What would be important to determine would be the degree of your stress and whether you can cope with it yourself or would benefit from counseling. Sometimes menopause can act as a catalyst to set off a stress reaction when the more basic cause is a problem in another area of the woman's life. If this is the case, it would likely be a good time to get assistance to deal with the problems.

If, however, the stress is relatively minor and you can cope with it yourself, you may find some of these techniques might work for you:

- Relaxation tapes. There are many tapes available. Some have the sounds of nature that are generally associated with relaxation. Others are specifically designed to teach you how to relax the different parts of your body.
- Listen to the music you find most relaxing.
- Take a long, relaxing bath.
- Yoga is a good combination of both exercising and relaxing.
- Get a massage.
- The use of positive imagery. Sit in a quiet spot by yourself, close your eyes and imagine a scene that is very positive and relaxing for you. It could be walking along a beach or sitting in front of a fireplace with a roaring fire and your favorite music in the background or it could be recollecting a pleasant memory.
- Relaxation breathing. Breathe from deep in your abdomen and count the length of time you inhale and exhale. The length of your inhalation should be shorter than your exhalation.
- You could take the problem that is causing your stress and reframe it by thinking about some positive aspects rather than focusing on the negative ones. Sometimes we can start to unrealistically interpret the positive and negative things in our lives and only emphasize the negative aspects. We can often in this process forget that there are any positive things. We all need to have a balanced view of life and it is very easy for the balance to go out of kilter when we have a great deal with which to cope.
- Exercise is an excellent way to get rid of stress as well as keeping yourself in better condition. Choose the type of exercise that best meets your own health needs. For some, a rigorous game of tennis may be beneficial. For others, walking may serve the same purpose.
- You may find there is some way to change the situation around you which will reduce the stress, e.g., start to express your feelings or anger.

Women's roles and menopause
Some researchers have found that women who work report fewer menopausal symptoms. While it is difficult to know how widespread these results might be, it does raise the question of how

women's roles may be related to how they experience menopause. It is very possible that it does not make a difference whether a woman works, or volunteers her time or has hobbies which she does at home or is a homemaker. What is probably more important is how the woman sees herself and whether she enjoys the roles she has. If she does, she will no doubt have a sense of competence and self-esteem which will make going through any experience easier. She will also focus more of her attention on other tasks than on her own symptoms.

In coping with menopause, it would no doubt be of help to a woman to evaluate her roles and determine how satisfying they are. A woman would also be wise to set goals for herself that are realistic and enjoyable.

The role of support groups

Over the past few years, support groups have been set up for menopausal women. They are based on the philosophy of women helping and supporting other women. It provides an opportunity for women to share their feelings and experiences during menopause and to discover that other women feel and experience the same things. For some women being part of a support group is a powerful and reinforcing situation. An excellent example of how effective a support group can be and in what ways they can be supportive is in a quote in *New Our Bodies, Ourselves*:

> "I had never been in any kind of support group before. I thought it would be a discussion group and everyone would be an expert except me, and I'd be embarrassed because I wasn't an expert on anything. But that's not the way this group worked. There's a lot of mutual help; people really listen to each other and laugh a lot. Now I don't worry about menopause or growing older the way I used to.
>
> "Validated by the new knowledge that I had the same powerful physical and emotional experiences as all women, I was proud to have gone through menopause and some difficult life changes at the same time. For instance, creating a new life for myself after my divorce. I love my friends and know they have gone through similar challenges."

Obviously this woman found a support group an excellent way to help her cope with menopause. From my discussions with women, they have described the feelings of pride, self-esteem, and support that they have developed from being in a support group. However, there are those who like privacy and feel more comfortable discussing their reactions to menopause on a one-to-one basis rather than in a group situation. If you are the kind of a person who would profit from being a member of a group of menopausal women, you could probably locate the nearest group through your local newspaper, women's clubs, Y.W.C.A., or church groups.

Evaluating information on menopause

It is becoming easier to find articles on menopause in popular magazines and newspapers. However, before applying the statements in the article to yourself, you may want to consider the following:

- The size of the group included in the article may be relatively small and, therefore, may not represent generally how the majority of women think, feel or behave.
- The conclusions reached in the article may differ depending on when the researchers consider menopause to happen: some call a woman menopausal when she has gone for three months without having a menstrual period, others use six months, and still others one or two years.
- Some of the conclusions have been based on information collected from women attending a clinic for their menopausal symptoms. The symptoms these women report may not reflect those of women who do not attend clinics.
- When reading about studies using measurements of estrogen, the findings may not be accurate due to the limited testing of the hormone. Estrogen levels tend to fluctuate, therefore it would be misleading to use only one measurement.
- If you read, for example, that there is a relationship between self-esteem and menopausal symptoms, you should realize this does not mean that there is a cause-and-effect relationship between the two, that is that self-esteem causes menopausal symptoms. There could be other factors that could affect both the level of self-esteem and menopausal symptoms, such as the support the woman has. Any behaviour is usually caused by many factors. Be suspicious if the study you are reading has looked at the effects of only one factor at a time. It is not unusual in the popular literature for information to be over-simplified and causal statements made when in fact they cannot be supported by the study.

As you can see, it is important not to jump to conclusions when reading any articles because there are many factors that can unintentionally mislead you.

Medication and menopause

As discussed earlier, there are different types of medication prescribed for women during menopause; hormones, anti-depressants, sleeping pills, and tranquilizers. Also, some women may use over-the-counter drugs to relieve some of their menopausal symptoms like sleeping problems or tension. The use of hormones has been extensively discussed in the last chapter and will not be referred to here. With respect to the other types of medication, before using any of them you may want to think about these points.

- Some researchers feel physicians believe menopause to be more traumatic than most women do. Therefore, some physicians may be prescribing medication unnecessarily. There are advantages to being actively involved in the decisions about the kinds of drugs you will take.
- Every woman differs in her ability to tolerate different types of drugs. You will need to monitor the effects of the drug on yourself and, if you feel the medication is bothering you in some way or is not helping you, this information should be given to your physician.
- Some women are allergic to a type of drug. Again, it reinforces the importance of self awareness and informing your doctor about your reactions to all treatment.
- You can develop a physical dependence on some drugs, which means that your body can then only function normally if you continue to use the drug. If you are physically dependent on a drug, when you stop using it you will experience withdrawal. That means without the drug, you may go through a number of different symptoms, ranging from mild to intense forms of discomfort.
- Other drugs may produce what is called psychological dependence. With psychological dependence you have an intense craving for the drug and feel you can not cope without it.
- Many of the tranquilizers, such as valium, can, if used for a long period of time, become physically and psychologically addictive. Regular use also creates tolerance, making it necessary to take more medication to achieve the required effect.
- Each of the different types of medication have their own side effects. For example, the side effects of valium include drowsi-

ness, dizziness, blurred vision, vertigo, headaches, impairment of memory, confusion, and depression. This does not mean that everyone who uses valium will become dependent on it nor that they will have the side effects. But some do. Ask your physician what the side effects are of any of the drugs you are prescribed.

- Alcohol is also a drug. In fact, the statistics show that it is the drug used most frequently by the majority of people. With alcohol you can develop a tolerance, making you feel you can drink more and more. You can also develop a psychological and physical dependence.

- Many drugs become potentially dangerous when they are mixed with each other. For example, you should avoid mixing alcohol and valium. When a physician prescribes a drug for you, make sure you tell him/her about any other drugs you are using. Again, do not assume he/she will remember.

- If you are using over-the-counter drugs, you would be wise to read the labels carefully to ensure the drug does not include a substance to which you are allergic or should not be taking for some other health-related reason. Do not just assume that because these drugs are so readily available they could not be potentially harmful to you. You can also become psychologically dependent on these types of drugs if you use them frequently enough.

- Sometimes the use of drugs can mask problems that should be dealt with more directly. For example, rather than simply giving an anti-depressant for depression, it may be wise, if it is likely that there are many reasons for the depression in addition to menopause or if the depression is long-standing, to get counseling.

- For most of the conditions for which you would be prescribed medication, there are other types of treatment available. When a doctor prescribes a drug for you, you would be wise to ask what other kinds of treatment might be available. If your physician has no other alternatives, you might ask for a second opinion.

Medication can be very helpful for some women, assisting them in coping with their menopausal symptoms. But medication can also be potentially harmful if not closely monitored and used appropriately.

Chapter Seven

Questions and Answers

In my discussions with women, there were many general questions they raised about menopause. This chapter will answer some of those questions.

Is there a lessening of sex drive with menopause?
One of the myths that has been perpetuated over the years is that menopausal women are no longer interested in sex. Actually, women's responses to sex after menopause are as varied as they were prior to this event. As Drs. Robert Greenblatt and Donald Perez have stated: "The rekindling or awakening of sexual excitement that occurs during the menopause and postmenopausal years frequently allows women, frigid in their earlier sexual experiences, to become sexually sensitive and interested. For others, however, the menopause with its waning hormonal levels, brings on a train of psycho-sexual disorders marked by a loss of sexual desire; depression and insecurity in the role as a sexual partner."

There have even been a series of studies carried out to try to determine more precisely women's attitudes to sex after menopause. These studies have basically tried to answer two questions: Does a woman's sex drive change after menopause? and, Is there a change in a woman's satisfaction during sex?

One American survey reported that approximately 60 percent of menopausal women had an unaltered sex drive, about 20 percent increased, and another 20 percent reported a decrease in their interest in sex. Other studies indicate other results, such as 50 percent of women showing a reduction in interest and 50 percent with no such reduction. Some researchers found that for some women, while the frequency of activity was the same, the types of sexual activities changed, e.g., less intercourse but the same amount of physical affection, manual genital-oral behaviours, and mutual masturbation. Others who were less active were significantly lower on all activities except affection. It is difficult to know exactly what causes the different results among studies. What we do know, however, is that as Drs. Kinsey, Masters, and Johnson indicated there is no limit with advancing years to female sexuality. According to these authors, it is possible and desirable to have sex well past age 60. In fact, Drs. William Masters and Virginia Johnson felt that women reached erotic peak in middle age and the sexual capabilities of women did not decline until late in life. They stated that women are fully capable of sexual performance at an orgasmic response level until well into their 80s, if regularly exposed to effective sexual stimulation. But, fewer women are sexually active after age 60.

A decline in sexual intercourse is not unusual for both women and men as they become older. It is important to remember that while the desire for, or frequency of, sexual intercourse may change with age, it may not diminish in pleasure. Many menopausal women who reported a decline in the frequency of sexual intercourse were happy with their sex life.

Again, the level of desire, frequency of sexual intercourse, attitude, and pleasure associated with sexuality is a very individual matter, both before and after menopause. Regardless of whether a woman experiences changes in her sexual desires and activities, the critical factor is how she feels about herself and her relationship with her husband/partner.

One additional question that many women raise with regard to sexuality is *the effect of a hysterectomy on sexual pleasure*. It is clear that having a hysterectomy need not affect a woman's sexual pleasure. In fact, for some women the operation eliminates some of the problems that previously affected their sex lives and after the hysterectomy their sex lives improve. One research study suggests that somewhere between 25 and 45 percent of women will notice a difference in their sexual arousal after the operation.

In the *New Our Bodies, Ourselves*, the Boston Women's Collective offers some explanations for the changes in sexuality, if they occur, after a hysterectomy.

- "Many women experience orgasm primarily when the penis or a lover's fingers push against the cervix and uterus, causing uterine contractions and increased stimulation of the abdominal lining (peritoneum). Without the uterus or cervix, there may be much less of this kind of sensation."

- "If the ovaries are removed, ovarian androgens which affect sexuality may be greatly reduced thus lowering sexual response. These hormones cannot be replaced by ERT. Even when the ovaries are not removed, this hormonal change may occur because the surgery may interfere with the blood supply."
- "Vaginal lubrication tends to lessen after oophorectomy" (removal of the ovaries).
- "Local effects of surgery may occasionally cause problems. If your vagina has been shortened. . . intercourse may be uncomfortable. Scar tissue in the pelvis or at the top of the vagina from either the vaginal or abdominal procedure can also cause painful intercourse."

Another cause of possible changes in sexuality after a hysterectomy is related by some to the symbolic meaning of the uterus. If a woman considers herself to be less feminine following the operation, it may interfere with her sexuality.

If your sexual desire is less around the time of menopause, it may help to be aware that this change is not abnormal nor necessarily due to your psychological adjustment; and recognize some of the reasons for this change and decide if this is what you want. If not, it may be the time to see your physician, if the cause is physical, that is, due to painful intercourse or problems with vaginal lubrication. On the other hand, it may be the time to re-examine your relationship with your sexual partner.

Menopause may be a good time to become more aware of yourself as a sexual being. If your pattern of sexuality synchronizes with your partner's and pleases both of you — no problem! However, if your partner's desire is greater than yours, it may give you an opportunity to improve your communication and solve the problem together. If your desire is greater than your partner's, you may need other outlets to satisfy yourself, such as masturbation.

Is there a relationship between menopause and heart disease?
There is considerable debate on the relationship between menopause and heart disease. Some researchers feel that the rate of heart disease increases for both men and women as they age, but throughout middle age there is a greater chance that men will

suffer a heart attack than women. Also some feel that if you control for age, the probability of a coronary heart attack is similar for both pre- and postmenstrual women.

The popularly accepted view is that menstruation, with higher levels of estrogen, protects women from coronary heart disease. For example, Judith Hill reported a study which acknowledged an "increase in coronary heart disease incidents which occurs by a sudden escalation in risk at the time of menopause."

Drs. Meeks and Bates feel that atherosclerosis (a disease in which fatty deposits develop on the inner walls of the arteries) is probably related to certain "serum lipid profiles." High concentrations of low density lipoproteins, they indicated, are linked to increased rates of atherosclerosis coronary vascular disease. On the other hand, concentrations of high density lipoproteins offer some protection to the disease. They also noted that there were lipid changes that occurred in menopausal women, with an increase in low density and decrease in high density lipoproteins. There are, however, other researchers who feel that susceptibility to coronary vascular disease is a result of a complex interaction between high lipids and age, menstrual status, weight gain, smoking, and amount of exercise.

Another factor that may be related to suceptibility of heart disease is the age at which menopause occurs. Drs. Meeks and Bates reported that women who have their ovaries removed prior to the age of 40, or who lose ovarian function prior to that age for some other reason, show an increased incidence of coronary heart disease.

This topic is a very complex one. More research is required before any definitive answer can be given. But it is clear that as women age, it becomes increasingly beneficial for them to watch their diet (eating foods that have high density lipoproteins and avoiding those with low density lipoproteins. Information about the content of food can be obtained from food guides); exercise regularly and appropriately for their age group; and avoid smoking, particularly if they are, based on their family history or health status, high risk for heart disease.

Can I become pregnant after menopausal symptoms have started?
Yes, it is possible to become pregnant during the perimenopausal stage. Even though your menstrual periods may be irregular and you may have even stopped menstruating for a few months, there is still a chance you can become pregnant. Some feel that contra-

ception should be used until you have stopped menstruating for at least a year.

According to Dr. Janet McArthur, "While conception is thus possible after menopause, pregnancies are rare. Fertility begins to decline more than a decade before the climacteric; only 1.6 percent of confinements occur in women over 40 and only 0.2 percent in women over 48 years of age. The decline was formerly attributed mainly to anovulation. However, recent studies show that women who are cycling regularly within the range of 21 to 35 days will ovulate during almost every cycle, regardless of their chronologic age."

It is recommended that women over the age of 35 or 40 do not use birth control pills for contraception, since the risks of high blood pressure, clot formation, and heart attacks increase with age. Thus, other forms of contraception should be used until it has been 12 months since your last period. It would be important to discuss with your physician the method of contraception that would be best for you. In addition, to reducing the chances of becoming pregnant, you will probably feel more relaxed in coping with missed periods if you are using a form of contraception.

How does a hysterectomy affect menopause?
There seem to be misconceptions about the relationship between hysterectomies and menopause. For example, many of the women to whom I spoke who had had a hysterectomy felt they would not go through menopause. This is not an unusual conclusion. In fact, the effect of a hysterectomy on menopause will depend on the type of operation a woman has had.

Hysterectomies are one of the most frequent major operations carried out in North America. Dr. Susanne Morgan stated that about half of the women in the United States would have a hysterectomy by the age of 65 and about 40 percent of those by the age of 40. While the statistics vary slightly, there seems to be a general agreement that a high percentage of women undergo this form of surgery. Statistics suggest that hysterectomies are performed considerably less frequently in Europe. Dr. van Keep and his colleagues, in a recent article, reported the occurrence of hysterectomies in six European countries (Belgium, France, West Germany, The Netherlands, Italy, and the United Kingdom). The percentages of hysterectomies ranged from 8.5 percent in France to 15.5 percent in Italy. Although even in Europe, where the frequency of the operation was less, there had been an increase in the incidence of this form of surgery between 1960 and 1980.

It seems that two of the earliest gynecological and surgical procedures were ovariectomy (removal of the ovaries) and clitoidectomy (removal of the clitoris). Dr. Anne Kasper described that these operations were prescribed for a number of disorders such as hysteria, nervousness, frigidity, masturbation, and to curb sexual excesses. According to Drs. Kincey and McFarlane, the earliest hysterectomy was performed by Dr. Blundell in Britain in 1828. With these early operations no form of anaesthetic was used. Since that time not only have the numbers increased and the reasons for the operation changed but also the techniques have improved.

In *The New Our Bodies, Ourselves*, the authors described graphically the different types of hysterectomies. Their diagram is, I think, extremely helpful for our understanding of the operation and I have included a copy of it here. As you can see in the diagram,

- A *partial hysterectomy* refers to the removal of the uterus — "After surgery the cervix and the stump of the uterus remain, requiring regular Pap tests."
- A *total hysterectomy or complete hysterectomy* involves the removal of the uterus and cervix. — "You will continue to ovulate but will no longer have menstrual periods; instead the egg is absorbed by the body into the pelvic cavity."
- A total hysterectomy with either the unilateral (one side) or bilateral (both sides) removal of the ovaries is called a *total hysterectomy with unilateral or bilateral oophorectomy*. Usually with this operation the fallopian tubes are also removed. If one ovary is removed you will still ovulate with the other one. If both are excised, you will obviously stop ovulating immediately.
- An *oophorectomy* means the removal of the ovary, either unilateral or bilateral. — "When both ovaries are removed, a hysterectomy is usually performed at the same time. Common reasons for oophorectomy include ectopic pregnancy [a pregnancy where the fertilized egg becomes lodged outside the uterus, usually in the fallopian tubes], endometriosis [the presence of the kind of lining usually in the uterus on the ovary], benign or malignant tumors or cysts on the ovary and pelvic inflammatory disease."

SOME COMMON AND UNCOMMON HEALTH AND MEDICAL PROBLEMS

Hysterectomy Procedures

These are the common procedures for hysterectomy. Rather than simply accepting the *name* of the procedure your surgeon proposes, ask for a complete description with diagram.

- *Total hysterectomy*, sometimes called *complete hysterectomy*. The surgeon removes the uterus and cervix, leaving the fallopian tubes and ovaries. You will continue to ovulate but will no longer have menstrual periods; instead the egg is absorbed by the body into the pelvic cavity.

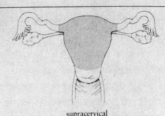

supracervical

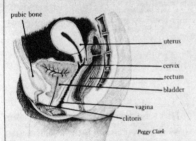

pubic bone

uterus
cervix
rectum
bladder
vagina
clitoris

Peggy Clark

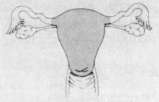

total or complete

PARTIAL HYSTERECTOMY *(uterus tipped to show line of surgical incision; ovary hidden). After surgery the cervix and the stump of the uterus remain, requiring regular Pap tests.*

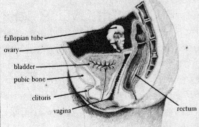

fallopian tube
ovary
bladder
pubic bone
clitoris
vagina
rectum

Peggy Clark

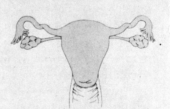

total with bilateral salpingo-oophorectomy

COMPLETE HYSTERECTOMY. *Removal of complete uterus, including cervix (ovaries and tubes are attached to top of vagina).*

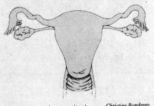

radical   *Christine Bondante*

Hysterectomies can either be abdominal or vaginal. With an abdominal hysterectomy, an incision is made in your abdomen. "The surgeon will have to recommend an abdominal incision if your ovaries are to be removed, if there is a large tumor in your uterus or if you have chronic pelvic disease. . . . However, in an abdominal hysterectomy they are more likely to remove healthy ovaries because they are accessible." With a vaginal hysterectomy the uterus is removed through the vagina. The incision is made inside the vagina.

With regard to menopause, as long as one of the ovaries remains, you will go through menopause. There has been some discussion about the timing of this event, but most seem to agree that menopause will occur at the time when you would have ordinarily gone through the process. But if both of your ovaries are removed, you will go through menopause right after surgery. Hot flashes are usually the first symptom women have, although some women might not have any symptoms.

Will I lose my femininity when I become menopausal?
We all have our own views of what femininity is. For many of us our definition is, at least partly, culturally determined. It can refer to a behavior, appearance or roles that we associate with being female. Maggie Scarf, in her book *Unfinished Business: Pressure Points in the Lives of Women,* discussed what is considered, in our culture, to be normally feminine behaviour. She suggested that normally feminine behaviour was associated with dependence, seeking approval of others, not being self sufficient, and defining success as pleasing others. She felt that a woman was considered to be unfeminine if she was competitive, ambitious, adventurous, not at all interested in appearance, aggressive, or assertive. Lillian Rubin, in *Women of a Certain Age,* also referred to competence not being considered to be an important goal for the feminine woman. With regard to appearance, what is considered feminine is defined for us by the media. In the media are portrayed the "ideal" for being feminine in attractiveness, skin care, hairstyle, makeup, clothing, and body type.

If one looks at the roles associated with femininity, the reproductive one is of prime importance. Femininity seems to be associated with being a good mother.

There are culturally-defined norms or expectations about what is considered to be feminine. Some women accept these norms while others do not. With menopause, there are changes that affect a woman's ability to reproduce. With declining estrogen levels, there are also changes in skin tone, fat distribution, and firmness of the breasts. The question is, are these changes really related to being feminine? For some women, they are; for others they are not. For still others, menopause can be a time when they reanalyze what femininity is, and redefine it as being "what, as a female, I am and I do." As discussed earlier, many women feel that being middle-aged, they now have the time to think about themselves and their own growth.

In *Passages*, Gail Sheehy referred to the writings of psychoanalyst Carl Jung who "was the first major analytic thinker to view middle life as the time of maximum potential for personality growth. We yearn at that time for the undividedness of self that has always been lacking. As the hope of finding security in another vanishes, the conflict is brought to a head. Consequently, many of our archetypal images of 'feminine' and of 'masculine', images we unconsciously project upon a mate, can be withdrawn. Jung talks about the necessity to 'confront our own contrasexual aspect' and to integrate it, which makes possible an extraordinary enrichment of all experience."

What is premature menopause?

Premature menopause is the term used to refer to the early permanent cessation of menstruation. Ages 35 or 40 are usually used as the cut cutoff point. According to Janice Delaney, Mary Jane Lupton and Emily Toth, it is experienced by about eight percent of women. They stated that the earliest case on record was of a nine-year old girl. They also described a case, reported by a 19th-century gynecologist, of a girl who had her first menstruation at age nine, was married at fifteen and a half and became menopausal at seventeen years.

It is necessary to differentiate premature menopause from long periods of amenorrhea (the stopping of menstrual periods), which can result from stress, severe dieting, exercising, or illness. Premature menopause is identifiable by an increase in the levels of the pituitary hormones.

Drs. Cutler and Garcia described some of the causes of premature menopause as genetic predilection or ovarian failure due to an autoimmune reaction secondary to rheumatic fever or inflammatory infections, such as mumps, affecting the ovaries. The surgical removal of the ovaries could be another possible cause.

Will other people know if I'm menopausal?
Some women are concerned that other people will know that they are in the perimenopausal stage. In fact, at least in the beginning of this stage, only you will know for sure. Others may feel that if you are depressed or excessively and unexpectedly irritable with no apparent cause, and you are in the age range where it is a possibility, that you are menopausal. Sometimes they may assume you are menopausal when you are not and sometimes it will be the other way around. Hot flashes may or may not be apparent to others. There have been times, while talking to women about menopause, where they have looked in the mirror and commented on how visible their hot flash was, when I did not notice the difference. Some women have found, when they looked in the mirror, that their hot flash is actually attractive. Others may actually be admiring your skin tone during your hot flash. Regardless of whether or not your symptoms are obvious, it is best just to be concerned about your own reactions and not try and interpret those of others.

Is there any way I can prepare my husband and children for my menopause?
Each one of us establishes with our family our own pattern of communication. Some women tend to be more open and others more reticent, protecting their families from their feelings or problems. Perhaps, as we become menopausal, it is a good time to re-evaluate the communication we do have and determine if we want to change it. For example, some women indicated that they discussed their symptoms, concerns or feelings about menopause with their families while others did not. Some know how their families felt about menopause while others were unfamiliar with their families' attitudes.

Some of the ways that might help in preparing your family for your menopause could be:

- to maintain open communications with your family so that when topics like menopause arise they can be discussed with comfort;
- to share information that you have on the topic with your family so they will not be as likely to accept societal myths;
- to share your feelings about menopause with your family so they can be more understanding
- discuss issues as they arise, for example, your son saying this his friend's mother must be menopausal because she is so irritable.

Is there anything I can do in earlier life to make my menopausal years easier?
There are many things that are of importance earlier in your life that can affect how you react to menopause.

- *A good diet* — research has shown that what you eat when you are younger can affect your peak bone mass that is so important in helping to prevent osteoporosis. A good diet is one that is high in calcium and low in protein.
- *Learning about menopause,* through reading and discussions can provide you with information that can affect your attitude and feelings to menopause.
- *Becoming aware of techniques to cope with stress,* such as yoga, abdominal breathing, and positive imagery, and *unpredictability,* such as learning how to look at alternative explanations, being more open to new situations and flexible in how you deal with them, can facilitate dealing with any potentially stressful situation.
- *Stop smoking* or smoke as little as possible.
- *Moderate alcohol consumption* is a good goal.
- A *regular exercise program,* established when you are younger, will be beneficial to you during your menopause and is easier than trying to set up a program when you are older.

Will menopause affect my personality and ability to work?
As mentioned earlier, the symptoms women experience during menopause vary in their number, type, intensity, frequency, and duration. Also, women's reactions to what can appear to be similar symptoms can be different. Drs. Mary and Michael Dosey noted that "for some women menopause may be a topic of intimacy, embarrassment or stigma. Some women may minimize or deny problems, while others may exaggerate them. For most women, despite some unpleasant reactions, the climacterium is not a crisis." For the majority of women, any changes, if they occur at all, in their personality and ability to work will be minor. Some women may find they feel more irritable or anxious and concentration may be minimally affected by menopausal symptoms. However, most researchers state that there is no specific constellation of psychiatric symptoms characteristic of menopause. Also, women during menopause, while they may feel depressed, are not at higher risk for a depressive disorder. Therefore, in general, any changes that may occur will be minimal. But

there are some women who either experience more intense symptoms or who, due to their personality, life style or physical health, are more vulnerable to symptoms. Some of these women may find that they are sufficiently depressed, anxious or irritable that it is interfering with their life and they require treatment. We still do not understand enough about menopause to know precisely how the biological (lower levels of estrogen or higher levels of the pituitary hormones) and the social/psychological (personality prior to menopause, social relationships, events occurring in their lives) changes contribute to the symptoms a woman experiences. But there are different types of treatment that can help women when the menopausal symptoms start to interfere with their life.

If I had trouble with my menstrual periods, will I also have a difficult menopause?

There are four types of menstrual problems that have been related to symptoms and the time of onset of menopause: dysmenorrhea (painful menstruation); amenorrhea (cessation of menstrual periods); menorrhagia (excessive flow of menses); premenstrual syndrome (PMS). Dr. Norris, in his book *PMS Premenstrual Syndrome*, described the following symptoms for PMS: irritability, tension, headache, depression, fatigue, breast swelling and tenderness, abdominal bloating, weight gain, increased thirst or appetite, cravings for sweet or salty foods, acne, asthma, and constipation. Other symptoms that he also felt could occur on a regular cyclical basis included such things as boils, herpes, hives, epilepsy, and migraines.

The research on menstrual problems and menopause is full of contradictions. Some feel that, for example, dysmenorrhea is related to menopausal distress. Some do not. From looking at the different studies, it is difficult to understand why some found a relationship while others did not. It is possible to conclude that for some women, the primary symptoms that were associated with their menstrual periods will become symptoms during the perimenopausal period. According to Dr. Norris, "most women with PMS find their symptoms end at or after menopause. . . . A small percentage of women who reach menopause or are postmenopausal do exhibit the cyclical and recurring symptoms. About ten percent of our patients have been through menopause but exhibit symptoms in a pattern that matches their earlier menstrual cycles. . . . Some women suffer worse PMS symptoms in the pre-menopause years. We have also seen a few women whose

PMS begins at menopause. It usually becomes clear that they had mild PMS prior to menopause, became worse with menopause and worsened after. But some really do suffer the onset at menopause. The symptoms tend to be irritability, vague muscle and joint aches, fatigue, lack of concentration, and sometimes excessive use of alcohol. Some doctors who diagnose PMS at this stage treat the menopause in a cycle of progesterone and estrogen. . ." We need much more research before we will be able to understand exactly the relationship between menstrual problems and menopause.

What can I do to prepare for menopause?
Probably the best way to be prepared is to be well informed about menopause. There are several sources from which you can get information: books and articles, your physician, support groups, to name just a few. It might be very helpful for you to get this information in advance so that you are reassured that any symptoms you have will be temporary. Also, it could be beneficial to know what treatment possibilities are available to you, and for what types of symptoms, so you can make decisions that will be best suited to your needs. In addition, it will help to share your experiences and feelings with others as they occur. As noted before, keeping track of your menstrual periods and any menopausal symptoms as they occur will make it easier to identify when changes are occurring. Understanding yourself and your body is an important part of your preparation for menopause.

Is there a male menopause?
Many terms have been used to describe changes that occur in some men during midlife (male menopause, midlife crisis, male climacteric). If you think about it, male menopause is a rather strange phrase to use, since menopause refers to the cessation of menstruation. Perhaps for men the change is symbolic.

The symptoms that have been associated with male menopause include irritability, anxiety, depression, fatigue, and inexplicable behaviour such as giving up responsibility (men may leave their wives and family or give up a position at work that they have seemed to enjoy for many years and search for a new life). It is identified by many as a time when men buy new sportscars, adopt a different style of dress, or marry a younger woman.

When I asked a group of women whether they felt men went through a change of life, only a couple of them said they did not think so or they really did not know. The majority of women agreed that men experienced something comparable to menopause.

- "The age varies. They think they are getting past their prime and they have missed out on life so they frantically make changes to make up for lost time."
- "It occurs in the mid-to late forties in the form of re-evaluation of their life and their achivements and deciding where to go from that point."
- "They get a little moody."
- "They become crazy and want to feel very young again. They feel they haven't achieved what they should have, they want to change mates and have fast cars and fancy clothes. They think their wives are getting old and they are not."
- "Probably in late 40s and 50s, when he thinks youth is gone, he may be attracted to younger women to give himself a lift. He worries if on occasion he is unable to have sexual intercourse due to impotency."

According to Mike Featherstone and Mike Hepworth, interest in the problems of the middle-aged man developed at the end of the last century. Their research indicated that the most explicit example of this concern was stated in a book by Sylvanus Stall, called *What a Man Of 45 Ought to Know*. Marie Stopes, the first authority in Britain on birth control, writing after the First World War, noted that she received many letters which described a condition similar to the symptoms of the male menopause. More recently, descriptions of life for the middle-aged man have included such terms as "a disastrous watershed for twentieth-century man" and the "malaise of our time." There have been articles and books written about the topic and conferences held.

It is very difficult to determine how widespead male menopause is since what we know about the symptoms of male menopause has been collected by therapists who are seeing middle-aged men who have problems. How representative this sample is of most men is unknown. Featherstone and Hepworth, in an article written in 1985, outlined a report by a therapist who estimated that only approximately 20 percent of Western male population avoid "the distressing effects of male menopause." On the other hand, Drs. Michael Farrell and Stanley Rosenberg, in a recent study on male menopause, found no evidence for a universal midlife crisis. They felt that men showed considerable variation in how they responded to being middle-aged.

Most researchers agree that the changes in sex hormones in men are very gradual. In order to understand some of the changes in sex hormones that occur with aging, you might be interested in how the male reproductive system works: The male reproductive system is also based on the complex interaction/feedback system between the hypothalamus and pituitary gland, which has been discussed before, and the testis, the male sex organ that produces the sex hormones. Many writers have stated that testicular functioning is primarily controlled by the two pituitary hormones, lutenizing hormone, and follicle stimula⁺ing hormone. In turn, the release of the two pituitary hormones is stimulated by the hormones from the hypothalamus, that is the gonadotrophin releasing hormone and lutenizing releasing hormone. Follicle stimulating hormone acts on the testis to initiate the development of sperm. Lutenizing hormone causes the cells in the testis to produce and secrete testosterone, the primary human androgenic hormone. Testosterone is responsible for sperm maturation. According to Dr. Howard Nankin, "Testosterone also has direct central nervous system actions, increasing sexual drive, potentiating the erectile reflex at both brain and spinal levels, and so altering tactile sensations in the genital area. Testosterone exerts negative feedback effects at both the hypothalamus and the pituitary, probably inhibiting the release of LRH (lutenizing releasing hormone) and of LH (lutenizing hormone) and of FSH (follicle stimulating hormone), thus helping to regulate its own production."

With aging, there is a slight increase in the lutenizing hormone and the follicle stimulating hormone, which becomes even higher in men over 70 years of age. The levels of testosterone also change slowly but they tend to become slightly less with aging. But according to Dr. Baker, "Few of the elderly men had testosterone levels below the normal range." He also reported that "there have been preliminary reports of longitudinal studies which do not show marked changes in elderly men (specially selected to exclude any illness) who have a female partner. Many subjects have hormone levels the same as those found in young men. However, many are younger (50 to 70 years) and could show changes in the future."

Dr. Baker stated "an altered response to gonadotrophin releasing hormone has been reported also, suggesting some resistance of the pituitary to the releasing hormone. Despite this, the high LH and FSH levels indicate that the main disorder in the age related decline in testicular function is a primary degeneration of the testis with reduced feedback inhibition of gonadotrophin secretion."

With regard to the changes in semen quality with age, again inconsistent findings have been reported. However, in general, it would appear that while there is some decline in sperm mobility with age, the majority of men can remain fertile for most of their lives. Dr. Nankin described a man who became a father when he was 94 years old.

There are a small number of men who do have a sex hormone deficiency. These deficiencies can cause a loss of interest in sex, inadequate or non-existent erections, and low semen count. Other signs include reduced growth of beard and body hair and a reduction in the size of the testes.

Most of the authorities feel that, in the majority of cases, sexual problems in men have a psychological or environmental cause. Some also suggest that stress may have an effect on the level of testosterone levels. However this conclusion needs further testing. Rosetta Reitz, in her book *Menopause: A Positive Approach*, also felt that sexual hormones could be affected by stress. She said, "I believe the degree of our stability, security, and self-confidence affects the way we respond to the amount of estrogen our bodies produce."

As in many other areas discussed in this book, there is still a need for considerable research before the contribution of physical factors to the changes in some men's behaviour at midlife can be fully understood. It would appear, however, that what is considered to be a "male menopause" is primarily based on psychological reasons. Some of the factors that may predispose a man to develop symptoms of male menopause are:

- bodily changes that come with aging (graying hair or loss of hair, wrinkles, changes in body proportion, increased weight);
- more limited maneuverability (age becomes more apparent when activities are restricted to younger people, at social clubs, for example);
- a heightened awareness of more limitations at work (fewer promotion prospects);
- ability to deal with stress. Drs. Farrell and Rosenberg have set up a typology to responses to midlife stress. They discuss four types of ways of dealing with situations. According to these authors:

– about 12 percent of men fall into the category of "anti-hero." These men are the ones who have a true middle-age identity crisis, which may be precipitated by a sudden crisis or may have more long-standing origins. Their characteristics include high degree alienation, active identity struggle, ego-oriented in their concerns, no interpersonal involvements, low in authoritarianism.

– approximately 32 percent fit the transcendent-generative category. This type of personality can assess his past and present and match them with his inner feelings to experience a conscious sense of satisfaction; few symptoms of distress; open to feelings; accepts out-groups and feels in control of his own fate.

– 26 percent fit the pseudo-developed category in which they are overtly satisfied, attitudinally rigid; deny their feelings; high in authoritarianism; high on covert depression and anxiety and high in symptom formation.

– the final group is approximately 30 percent of the male population and is called the punitive-disenchanted group. They are highest in authoritarianism; dissatisfaction associated with environmental factors; conflict with children.

According to Geoffrey Aquilina Ross, the author of a book *How To Survive the Male Menopause*, the major issue in male menopause is the need for fulfillment in a strictly personal way: some men are afraid of failure; others feel they are missing out; some become aggressive because of frustration; others complain that life seems to take on a negative form; some are irritable because of discontentment; some are panicked, and wake up at night with an image of failure or a sense of futility; lack of opportunity for further personal fulfilment, problems with sex, money or work; some are listless; others indecisive, bored, restless, self questioning; some daydream as a form of escapism; others become overly concerned about their health; some drink too much alcohol; and others think a divorce may help them start again.

There is no question that some men present themselves at their physician's, psychiatrist's or psychologist's office with an array of symptoms very similar to what has just been described. Many health care workers feel that the male menopause is a result of trying to come to terms with getting older.

When a group of women were asked whether their mates' change of life affected them, their views were mixed. Some felt male menopause would not affect them. Others felt it would be difficult if their husband "went on a youth kick"; "gets strange"; "has affairs"; or "if it troubles him." Many also said that just as they need understanding at middle-age, so do their husbands. In fact, recognizing the stresses on middle-aged people may help both the husband and wife to work together.

Chapter Eight

Menopause Can Be a Fulfilling Experience

We all experience menopause in our own individual way. Some of us look forward to menopause; some of us are anxious, and some of us have a combination of both positive and negative feelings. All of these states are understandable because it is a new experience that affects all women differently.

- "In discussion with friends regarding menopause, the most common feelings have been those of relief — finally no more menstruation. The problems are mostly those which occur at the onset of menopause — heavy and irregular bleeding. Several women have experienced symptoms. Not one has mentioned depression or related problems. I do not know of a single woman who does not look forward to menopause."
- "It is sometimes an uncomfortable experience. If you allow the symptoms to become so important, I believe it can make one a nervous wreck. I believe it is healthy and comforting to talk openly about it with your family, whether males or females so they understand your actions, e.g., when having a flush. When talking to other women and comparing symptoms it can be comforting to know yours is not the only body experiencing this phenomenon. Mental attitude is so important — to dwell on it would be devastating. It is a good time for women to go back into the work force to keep their minds busy on other things."

Understanding your menopausal symptoms will not cure them but it will help you to get through the experience. It should give you more confidence to know that there is increasingly more openness surrounding the topic of menopause. We are now starting to get rid of the myths that have defined what menopausal women should be. The symptoms need no longer be ignored. There are a variety of different types of treatment available and more being researched daily. As women become more receptive to their own needs, support groups have become an additional source of information and understanding. As one can see, it is important to let other people know what your needs are in order to fully benefit from the resources around you. Menopause can be a fulfilling experience. Perhaps the best way to get the most out of it is to feel confident about ourselves.

Selected Bibliography

Baker, H.W.G. "Is there a male menopause?" In *Australian Family Physician* (1984), 13, 726—728.

Bates, G. William. "On the Nature of the Hot Falsh." In *Clinical Obstetrics and Gynecology* (1981), 24, 231-241.

Brody, Jane E. *The New York Times Guide to Personal Health.* New York: Avon Books, 1982.

Casper, R.F. and S.S.C. Yen. "Neuroendocrinology of Menopausal Flushes: An Hypothesis of Flush Mechanism." In *Clinical Endocrinology* (1985), 22, 293-312.

Conway, Jim and Sally Conway. *Women in Mid-Life Crisis.* Wheaton: Tyndale House, 1983.

Cutler, Winnifred B. and Celso-Ramón Garcia. *The Medical Management of Menopause and Premenopause.* London: J.B. Lippincott Co., 1984.

Cutler, Winnifred B., Celso-Ramón Garcia, and David A. Edwards. *Menopause: A Guide for Women and the Men Who Love Them.* New York: W.W. Norton, 1983.

Dege, Kristi, and Jacqueline Gretzinger, "Attitudes of Families toward Menopause." In A. Voda, M. Dinnerstein, and S. O'Donnell (eds.), *Proceedings at the Third Menstrual Cycle Conference.* Austin: University of Texas Press, 1982, 60-69.

Delaney, Janice, Mary Jane Lupton and Emily Toth. *The Curse: A Cultural History of Menstruation.* New York: Dutton, 1976.

Farrell, Michael P., and Stanley D. Rosenberg. *Men at Mid-Life.* Boston: Auburn House, 1981.

Kaufert, P. "The Menopausal Woman and Her Use of Health Services." In *Maturitas* (1980), 2, 191-206.

Lanson, Lucienne. *From Woman to Woman: A Gynecologist Answers Questions about You and Your Body.* New York: Alfred A. Knopf, 1981.

Lock, Margaret. "Ambiguities of Aging: Japanese Experience and Perceptions of Menopause." In *Culture, Medicine and Psychiatry* (1986), 10, 23-45.

Lock, Margaret. "Models and Practice in Medicine: Menopause as Syndrome or Life Transition." In *Culture, Medicine and Psychiatry* (1982), 6, 261-280.

McArthur, Janet W. "The Contemporary Menopause." In *Primary Cure* (1981), 8, 141.

McKinlay, S.M., and J.B. McKinlay. "Selected Studies of the Menopause." In *Journal of Biosocial Science* (1973), 5, 533-555.

McKinlay, Sonja M., and Margot Jefferys. "The Menopause Syndrome." In *British Journal of Preventive and Social Medicine* (1974), 28, 108-115.

Meeks, G. Rodney and G. William Easing Bates. "The Climacteric." In *Medical Aspects of Human Sexuality* (1986), 20, 91-107.

Neugarten, Bernice L., Vivian Wood, Ruth J. Kraine, and Barbara Loomis. "Women's Attitudes toward the Menopause." In *Vita Humana* (1963), 6, 140-151.

Neugarten, Bernice L. and Gunhild O. Hagestad. "Age and the Life Course." In Robert H. Binstock and Ethel Shanas (eds.), *Handbook of Aging and the Social Sciences.* New York: Van Nostrand, 35-57.

Norris, Ronald V., with Colleen Sullivan. *PMS: Premenstrual Syndrome.* New York Rawson Associates, 1983.

Nutrition Almanac. Revised edition. New York: McGraw-Hill, 1979.

Perlmutter, Johanna F. "A Gynecological Approach to Menopause." In Malkah T. Notman and Carol C. Nodelson (eds.), *The Woman Patient: Medical and Psycholgical Interfaces*. New York: Plenum Press, 1978, 323-336.

Reitz, Rosetta. *Menopause: A Positive Approach*. New York: Penguin Books, 1979.

Reuben, David. *Everything You Always Wanted to Know about Sex*. New York: David McKay Co., 1969.

Ross, Geoffrey Aquilina. *How to Survive the Male Menopause*. London: Elm Tree Books, 1984.

Rubin, Lillian. *Women of a Certain Age: The Midlife Search for Self*. New York: Harper & Row, 1979.

Seaman, Barbara, and Gideon Seaman. *Women and the Crisis in Sex Hormones*. New York: Bantom Books, 1978.

Smith, Wendy, in consultation with Dr. Stanton Cohn. *Osteoporosis: How to Prevent the Brittle Bone Disease*. New York: Simon & Schuster, 1985.

Sontag, Susan. "The Double Standard of Aging." In S. Gordon (ed.), *Sexuality Today and Tomorrow* (1976), 350-366.

Soules, Michael R., and William J. Bremner "The Menopause and Climacteric: Endocrinologic Basis and Associated Symptomatology." In *Journal of the American Geriatrics Society* (1982), 30, 547-561.

Trien, Susan Flamholtz. *Change of Life: The Menopause Handbook*. New York: Ballantine Books, 1986.

Voda, Ann M. and Mona Eliasson. "Menopause: The Closure of Menstrual Life." In *Women and Health* (1983), 8, 137-156.

Voda, Ann M., with James Tucker. *Menopause: Me and You*. Salt Lake City: College of Nursing, 1984.

Weideger, Paula. *Menstruation and Menopause: The Physiology and Psychology, The Myth and the Reality*. New York: Alfred A. Knopf, 1980.

Wilson, Robert. *Feminine Forever*. New York: M. Evans & Co., 1966.

Index

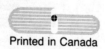

Printed in Canada